Advances in Anatomy, Embryology and Cell Biology
Ergebnisse der Anatomie und Entwicklungsgeschichte
Revues d'anatomie et de morphologie expérimentale

52/1

W0228178

Editors

A. Brodal, Oslo · W. Hild, Galveston · J. van Limborgh, Amsterdam · R. Ortmann, Köln
T. H. Schiebler, Würzburg · G. Töndury, Zürich · E. Wolff, Paris

Advances in Anatomy, Embryology and Cell Biology
Ergebnisse der Anatomie und Entwicklungsgeschichte
Revues d'anatomie et de morphologie expérimentale

Springer-Verlag Berlin Heidelberg GmbH

This journal publishes reviews and critical articles covering the entire field of normal anatomy (cytology, histology, cyto- and histochemistry, electron microscopy, macroscopy, experimental morphology and embryology and comparative anatomy). Papers dealing with anthropology and clinical morphology will also be accepted with the aim of encouraging co-operation between anatomy and related disciplines.

Papers, which may be in English, French or German, are normally commissioned, but original papers and communications may be submitted and will be considered so long as they deal with a subject comprehensively and meet the requirements of the "Ergebnisse".

For speed of publication and breadth of distribution, this journal appears in single issues which can be purchased separately; 6 issues constitute one volume.

It is a fundamental condition that submitted manuscripts have not been, and will not simultaneously be submitted or published elsewhere. With the acceptance of a manuscript for publication, the publishers acquire full and exclusive copyright for all languages and countries.

25 copies of each paper are supplied free of charge.

Les résultats publient des sommaires et des articles critiques concernant l'ensemble du domaine de l'anatomie normale (cytologie, histologie, cyto- et histochimie, microscopie électronique, macroscopie, morphologie expérimentale, embryologie et anatomie comparée. Seront publiés en outre les articles traitant de l'anthropologie et de la morphologie clinique, en vue d'encourager la collaboration entre l'anatomie et les disciplines voisines.

Seront publiés en priorité les articles expressément demandés, nous tiendrons toutefois compte des articles qui nous seront envoyés dans la mesure où ils traitent d'un sujet dans son ensemble et correspondent aux standards des «Ergebnisse». Les publications seront faites en langues anglaise, allemande et française.

Dans l'intérêt d'une publication rapide et d'une large diffusion les travaux publiés paraitront dans des cahiers individuels, diffusés séparément: 6 cahiers forment un volume.

En principe, seuls les manuscrits qui n'ont encore été publiés ni dans le pays d'origine ni à l'étranger peuvent nous être soumis. L'auteur s'engage en outre à ne pas les publier ailleurs ultérieurement.

Les auteurs recevront 25 exemplaires gratuits de leur publication.

Die Ergebnisse dienen der Veröffentlichung zusammenfassender und kritischer Artikel aus dem Gesamtgebiet der normalen Anatomie (Cytologie, Histologie, Cyto- und Histochemie, Elektronenmikroskopie, Makroskopie, experimentelle Morphologie und Embryologie und vergleichende Anatomie). Aufgenommen werden ferner Arbeiten anthropologischen und morphologisch-klinischen Inhaltes, mit dem Ziel, die Zusammenarbeit zwischen Anatomie und Nachbardisziplinen zu fördern.

Zur Veröffentlichung gelangen in erster Linie angeforderte Manuskripte, jedoch werden auch eingesandte Arbeiten und Originalmitteilungen berücksichtigt, sofern sie ein Gebiet umfassend abhandeln und den Anforderungen der „Ergebnisse" genügen. Die Veröffentlichungen erfolgen in englischer, deutscher und französischer Sprache.

Die Arbeiten erscheinen im Interesse einer raschen Veröffentlichung und einer weiten Verbreitung als einzeln berechnete Hefte; je 6 Hefte bilden einen Band.

Grundsätzlich dürfen nur Arbeiten eingesandt werden, die nicht gleichzeitig an anderer Stelle zur Veröffentlichung eingereicht oder bereits veröffentlicht worden sind. Der Autor verpflichtet sich, seinen Beitrag auch nachträglich nicht an anderer Stelle zu publizieren.

Die Mitarbeiter erhalten von ihren Arbeiten zusammen 25 Freiexemplare.

Manuscripts should be addressed to/Envoyer les manuscrits à/Manuskripte sind zu senden an:

Prof. Dr. A. BRODAL, Universitetet i Oslo, Anatomisk Institutt, Karl Johans Gate 47 (Domus Media), Oslo 1/Norwegen

Prof. W. HILD, Department of Anatomy. The University of Texas Medical Branch, Galveston, Texas 77550 (USA)

Prof. Dr. J. van LIMBORGH, Universiteit van Amsterdam, Anatomisch-Embryologisch Laboratorium, Amsterdam-O/Holland, Mauritskade 61

Prof. Dr. R. ORTMANN, Anatomisches Institut der Universität, D-5000 Köln-Lindenthal, Lindenburg

Prof. Dr. T. H. SCHIEBLER, Anatomisches Institut der Universität, Koellikerstraße 6, D-8700 Würzburg

Prof. Dr. G. TÖNDURY, Direktion der Anatomie, Gloriastraße 19, CH-8006 Zürich

Prof. Dr. E. WOLFF, Collège de France, Laboratoire d'Embryologie Expérimentale, 49 bis Avenue de la belle Gabrielle, Nogent-sur-Marne 94/France

M. Z. M. Ibrahim

Glycogen and its Related Enzymes of Metabolism in the Central Nervous System

With 13 Figures

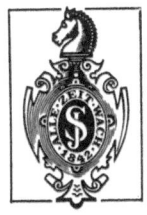

Springer-Verlag Berlin Heidelberg GmbH 1975

Dr. M. Z. M. Ibrahim
Department of Human Morphology
School of Medicine
American University of Beirut
Beirut, Lebanon

ISBN 978-3-540-07454-0   ISBN 978-3-642-86875-7 (eBook)
DOI 10.1007/978-3-642-86875-7

Library of Congress Cataloging in Publication Data. Ibrahim, Mohamed Z   M   Glycogen and its related enzymes of metabolism in the central nervous system. (Advances in anatomy, embryology, and cell biology; 52.1) Bibliography: p.   Includes index. 1. Glycogen metabolism. 2. Enzymes. 3. Central nervous system. I. Title. II. Series. [DNLM: 1. Brain—Metabolism. 2. Glycogen—Metabolism. 3. Glycogen phosphorylase. 4. Glycogen synthetase. W1 AD433k v. 52 fasc. 1/WL300 I14g] QL801.E67 vol. 52, fasc. 1 [QP702.G58] 574.4'08s [612'.814] 75-33065

Contents

1. Introduction

The glycogen content of normal mammalian CNS is small when compared with that of some other mammalian tissues such as liver and muscle. Nevertheless, this glycogen content normally comprises at least one quarter of its total reserve of energy, the rest being adenosine triphosphate (ATP), phosphocreatine and glucose. Since this glycogen undergoes a turnover 50–100 times that of brain lipids, and exceeds by several orders of magnitude that of liver glycogen, it most likely plays a dynamic role in the metabolism of brain, Gatfield *et al.* (1966), Prasannan and Subrahmanyam (1968b), Brunner *et al.* (1971), Edwards and Rogers (1972) and Watanabe and Passonneau (1973).

Glycogen also has an unequal distribution in the normal mammalian brain and spinal cord (Shimizu and Kumamoto, 1952; Shimizu and Okada, 1957; Friede, 1966; Shanthaveerappa *et al.*, 1966; Ibrahim *et al.*, 1970a), and it is possible that areas showing more glycogen "are inherently vulnerable and that their extra glycogen is an added protective mechanism" (Ibrahim, 1972). However, this is probably not the only explanation for the unequal distribution of glycogen since it is suggested for instance that neuronal glycogen may be normally implicated in the process of synaptic transmission (Shanthaveerappa *et al.*, 1966; Drummond and Bellward, 1970) and that retinal glycogen plays a role in the normal dark-light adaptation sequence (Shimizu and Maeda, 1953). Also, a wide variety of physiological, pathological and experimental conditions leads to a common response in the CNS, namely, accumulation of glycogen. A full comprehension of the mechanisms underlying such accumulation should assist in better understanding its function(s) and, possibly also, other aspects of CNS metabolism. Application is direct to problems in neurosurgery—in which trauma of the brain and oedema are an integral part—, to acute and delayed radionecrosis and to regional susceptibility of the CNS to various forms of hypoxia and intoxication.

In this communication we shall, therefore, briefly review some biochemical aspects of glycogen and its related enzymes (Fig. 1) and then review methods employed in the preservation of the normal distribution in the CNS of glycogen and also of phosphorylase (α-1,4-Glucan:orthophosphate glucosyl-transferase, E.C. 2.4.1.1) alone and in combination with branching enzyme (α-1,4-Glucan: α-1,4-glucan 6-glycosyl-transferase, E.C. 2.4.1.18), and of glycogen synthetase (UDP glucose:α-1,4-glucan, α-4-glucosyltransferase, E.C. 2.4.1.11). We shall then discuss some of the conditions in which excess of glycogen is found. From this discussion an attempt will be made to see if there is a common aetiology underlying the glycogen accumulation under various conditions.

2. Glycogen

2.1. Biochemical Considerations

This branched polyglucose is a storage form of readily available carbohydrate maximally stored in liver and muscle and, to a small extent, in CNS. It consists

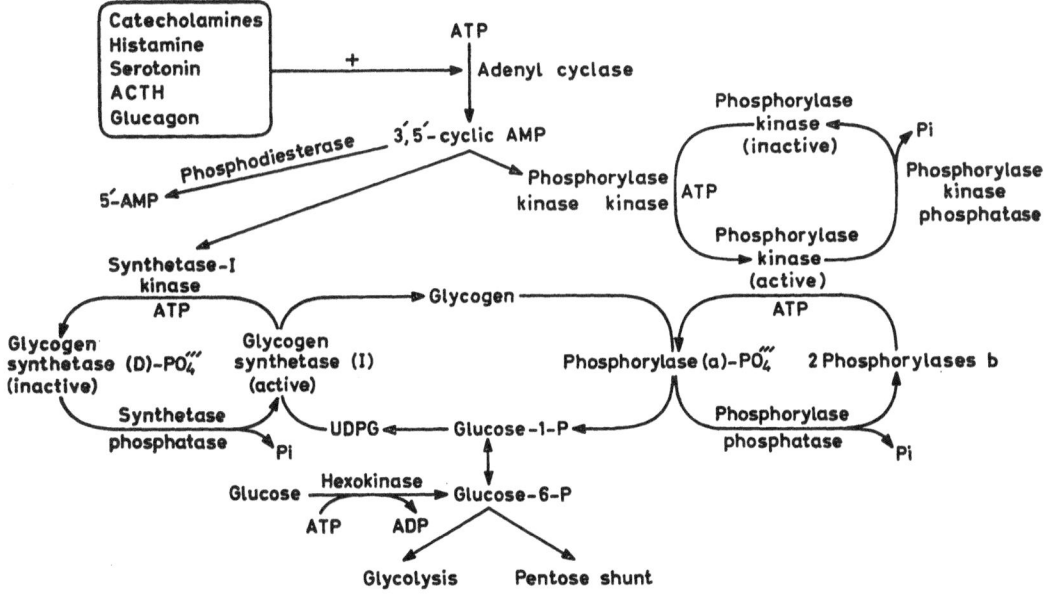

Fig. 1. A simplified schematic diagram representing some interactions of glycogen metabolism

of main (B) chains and side (A) chains with α-1 $\rightarrow$ 4-glucosidic linkages between the glucose molecules except at the points of origin of the side chains where the linkage is an α-1 $\rightarrow$ 6-glucosidic one (see e.g. Manners, 1968). It is readily hydrolysed in liver to glucose to maintain blood levels but, in muscle and CNS, glycogenolysis provides energy for local use only. It has traditionally been regarded by Biochemists as present in both "lyo" and "desmo" forms. The "lyo" form is that part which is extractable with cold trichloracetic acid, while the "desmo" form is that part which is not; the latter, however, is extractable with potassium hydroxide (Wanson and Drochmans, 1968; Leske and Mayersbach, 1969). Isolation of *particulate* glycogen from various sources was first achieved by Lazarow (1942). He demonstrated various size particles depending on the source but generally falling within two categories; this categorization is recognized now. There are large particles termed α-particles, with an average diameter of 1 000 Å— i.e. almost visible by light microscopy—and molecular weight of $100–400 \times 10^6$; and smaller ones, termed β-particles, with an average diameter of 300–400 Å and molecular weight of $4–10 \times 10^6$ (Revel, 1964; Drochmans and Dantan, 1968; Childress *et al.*, 1970; Smitherman *et al.*, 1972). Both these particles have been seen by electron microscopy (Revel, 1964; Wanson and Drochmans, 1968; Childress *et al.*, 1970; Bhagwat and Wong, 1972; de Bruijn, 1973); actually, the α-particles are conglomerations—generally rosette-shaped—of the smaller β-forms and are either free or related to profiles of endoplasmic reticulum. These β-particles were generally regarded as the ultimate unit until Drochmans and co-workers (Drochmans and Dantan, 1968; Wanson and Drochmans, 1968) and Childress *et al.* (1970), using extraction with potassium hydroxide, found that the smallest "subunits" of β-particles are only 150–220 Å with a molecular weight of $1–5 \times 10^6$.

7

It has been speculated that these "β-subunits" represent "the common unit for morphologists and biochemists" (Drochmans and Dantan, 1968).

Revel (1964) stressed that the α- and β-particles simply represent the extremes of a graded spectrum of particle sizes. These various particles presumably reflect different solubility patterns manifest during attempts at preserving them and/or reflect the nutritional and endocrinological states of the animal (Stetten and Stetten, 1960); these would directly govern the molecular weight upon which the solubility must partly depend (Tata, 1964; Leske and Mayersbach, 1969). This is not to suggest that protein related to these particles is all fixed from soluble cytoplasmic protein. Lazarow (1942) found that centrifuged unfixed particulate glycogen contains 92–93.5% carbohydrate and approximately 1% protein, the rest being water. He felt that this small amount of protein plays "a very important role in the maintenance of the complex" causing dispersed glycogen to become particulate. Wanson and Drochman's (1968) figure for this bound protein is 3% and Revel's (1964) findings suggest that it would not in fact play such an important role in granule synthesis and maintenance; Revel found that protein-free glycogen has the same appearance as that in situ. As a matter of fact the model drawn by French (1964) for the smallest glycogen particle, which he found has a diameter of about 360 Å, is that of a more-or-less spherical rebranched molecule and does not include internally located protein, but he does estimate a molecular weight for the particle of $4–10 \times 10^6$ if it is hydrated. This protein might represent then the enzymes of metabolism of glycogen which have been seen in intimate relationship with it.

2.2. Modes of Preservation

Fifty percent of muscle glycogen and 80% of liver glycogen is in soluble form—this is not synonymous with "lyo" form—the solubility being probably influenced by its molecular weight (Leske and Mayersbach, 1969). Also, postmorten glycogenolysis, induced by anoxia-stimulated phosphorylase activity, is very rapid (Hutchins and Rogers, 1970; Pontén et al., 1973). Hence, quantitative, in situ, preservation of glycogen requires very prompt handling.

Fixation

This is the method that is best suited to routine work on large blocks of tissue. The fixative should be rapidly penetrating and should produce a fine proteinaceous meshwork to trap the smallest particles of glycogen; "the particulate size of glycogen" is then also critical (Pearse, 1968, p. 89; Smitherman et al., 1972). According to these workers fixation of glycogen is only tenable through the first of the following three mechanisms generally thought to be operative:

a) Physical entrapment in a surrounding proteinaceous matrix (see also Leske and Mayersbach, 1969).

b) Binding to protein which when fixed renders the glycogen insoluble.

c) Dehydration resulting in decreased solubility (see also Pearse, 1968).

Although "fixation" of glycogen is, in fact, widely held to entail this physical entrapment in a protein meshwork yet, on histochemical grounds (Pearse, 1968) and on morphological ultrastructural grounds (Revel, 1964), this may not be true. Dehydration of glycogen particles by ethanol could render them insoluble as they become denatured, and fixation, even in formalin vapour, could induce linkages between the –OH groups of the polyglucose chains regardless of the presence of protein (Pearse, 1968, p. 89). Nevertheless, fixation for light microscopy in a mixture containing picric acid, which is a protein fixative that forms a fine meshwork coagulum (Smitherman et al., 1972), is still held to be the best for small blocks (Swigart et al., 1960; Cznarecki, 1971), as well as for sections (Swigart et al., 1960); unlike the findings of Smitherman et al. (1972) no glycogen was detected leaking into the fixing fluids (Cznarecki, 1971). Also the pH of the fixative is critical since acid fixatives tend to clump glycogen and, in electron microscopy, give pale and poorly defined granules (Bhagwat and Wong, 1972).

It is generally held that it is only the "lyo" fraction of glycogen that is demonstrable histochemically (see Pearse, 1968, p. 89), but as shown by the fixation experiments of Swigart et al. (1968) and Cznarecki (1971), very nearly all glycogen can be preserved and demonstrated. Leske and Mayersbach (1969) concur since they conclude that histochemically-demonstrable glycogen does not depend on the existence of two types of glycogen. In fact, they found that unfixed cryostat sections showed glycogen preservation best of all, this presumably being due to staining of *all* glycogen present.

Although all authors agree that that ethanol causes "glycogen flight" yet they advocate its use, provided it is combined with picrate. They also agree that in large blocks inactivation of hydrolytic enzymes in the more central parts is slow and hence glycogenolysis will occur there and cause artifactual loss of the polysaccharide. Furthermore, opinion is unanimous that the use of the fixative cold (4°C) should be the practice. Therefore, in all our studies on brain we have rapidly removed tissues (within 1–1^1/$_2$ min) from animals killed by exsanguination under light ether anaesthesia and fixed them immediately in cold Rossman's fluid for 24–48 hr. Ideally, quenching of blocks prior to immersion fixation (Leske and Mayersbach, 1969) or fixation by perfusion with cold Rossman's fluid (Shimizu and Kumamoto, 1952) should be done.

Several studies on the correlation between histochemical detection and tissue concentration of glycogen have been done. It was found that, using alcoholic fixatives (e.g. Carnoy) and periodic acid-Schiff (PAS) as the stain, the average general threshold for detection was 200 mg-% (see Pearse, 1968, p. 91); for myocardium it was 100 mg-% (Wittels, 1963). This limit to demonstrability, as well as the use of fixation procedures of varying effectiveness, accounts for discrepancies between the findings of different authors and especially between light and electron microscopic studies (see later).

Freeze-Drying and Freeze-Substitution

These techniques, at least on theoretical grounds, are generally held to be superior to fluid fixation procedures especially when the blocks are exposed to formaldehyde vapour. However, Swigart et al. (1960) have found that freeze-drying is no better than fixation in Rossman's fluid (see also Pearse, 1968, p. 91). Owing to their complexity and unproven superiority these techniques are not recommended for routine practice.

2.3. Histochemical Demonstration

Whatever the histochemical method employed for the detection of glycogen, control slides previously digested with salivary amylase, malt diastase or α- and β-amylase (Takeuchi, 1958) are essential especially when staining is done with PAS; several substances other than glycogen can be thus stained. The recognized techniques (Pearse, 1968, p. 363) include the iodine technique employed since the time of Claude Bernard; Best's ammoniacal carmine; the PAS sequence with various modifications; acid hydrolysis and oxidation followed by demonstration of revealed aldehyde groups by various silver solutions; fluorescence methods using periodic acid salicyloyl hydrazide sequence (Burns and Neame, 1966). All these techniques have their place but because the iodine and PAS techniques are pertinent to further discussion they will be mentioned in a little more detail.

The iodine technique employs Lugol's solution (I, 1 g: KI, 2 g: distilled water, 100 ml); its more diluted form (water, 300 ml) is Gram's iodine, which is still further diluted 1 in 10 with water for staining polyglucose products of enzymic activity (see p. 21). The advantage of this technique is the variability of colour obtained with different carbohydrate molecules. Thus glycogen gives a red-brown colour while shorter-chained and less-branched polyglucoses give different colours varying from greenish-blue to violet or reddish-purple. The disadvantages of this technique are its low specificity for glycogen, its rather indistinct localization and its fading with time even when special dehydrating and clearing techniques are employed. For staining experimentally-induced polyglucoses it has distinct advantages which will be mentioned later.

The PAS technique used as such, or as modified by Shimizu and Kumamoto (1952) by the use of lead tetra-acetate instead of periodate oxidation, is excellent for routine use on paraffin sections. Bulmer's (1959) sequence employs an aldehyde blockade step (by alcoholic dimedone) between periodic acid and the Schiff solution. This increases considerably the specificity of the technique for glycogen and experimentally-induced polyglucoses (see p. 21). This for us, has been the method of choice for routine work; the colour produced is strong, localization is excellent and there is no fading. Its disadvantage is related to the identification of experimental polyglucoses to be discussed presently.

2.4. Normal Distribution *

Because of the rapid activation of phosphorylase and the presence of other glycogenolytic enzymes (α-glucosidase and α-amylase), if not inhibited promptly by suitable fixation after death, glycogen of CNS normally disappears quickly, and in some places more so than others (see p. 8). Therefore, studies on the human topographical distribution are very difficult, and relatively accurate studies are limited to such animals as the cat, dog and the rodents in which age differences are seen as well. Thus in the newborn cat and dog the higher centers, viz. cerebral cortex and basal ganglia, contain more glycogen than in the adults

---

* Based on articles by Schabadasch (1939), Chesler and Himwich (1943), Shimizu and Kumamoto (1952), Shimizu and Maeda (1953), Oksche (1961), Kuwabara and Cogan (1961), Hutchinson and Kuwabara (1962), Niemi (1965), Friede (1966), Shanthaveerappa et al. (1966), Ibrahim et al. (1970a) Edwards and Rogers (1972) and Vigh-Teichmann and Vigh (1974).

whereas the reverse is the case for the cerebellum, medulla oblongata and spinal cord (Chesler and Himwich, 1943). However, a blanket statement is usually made that neonate and young animal brains contain much more glycogen, and have lower metabolic rates, than adults; both of these factors are usually held to account for the well-known relative resistence of such animals to anoxia and ischaemia (Edwards and Rogers, 1972).

Glycogen is demonstrable in the retinae of several species including man with an inverse relationship to the blood supply (see Niemi, 1965). It is located mainly in Müller's cells but some glycogen can be seen also in the photoreceptor cells, especially their outer segments, horizontal cells and, sometimes, in the ganglion cells. Dark-adapted retinae contain more than the light-adapted (Shimizu and Maeda, 1953), and according to Kuwabara and Cogan (1961) retinal glycogen is resistant to starvation.

Rich deposits are seen in the leptomeninges, the nerve fibre and neuroglia-ependymal layers of the olfactory bulb, the outer molecular layer and Hild's astroglial limiting layer of the cerebral cortex, especially around the lateral rhinal fissure and the pyriform cortex, and the molecular layer of the cerebellar cortex. Smaller amounts are seen in the connective tissue stroma of the choroid plexuses, and sometimes in its epithelium. Granules are abundant under the ependymal lining of the entire ventricular system, especially in the adjacent medial part of the caudate nucleus, but not in the ependymal cells themselves, except in the optic recess of the third ventricle. Moderate amounts occur in the subcommissural organ and large amounts in the hypothalamus, infundibulum and tuber cinerum especially in the ependymal fibers. Scanty deposits are found in the molecular layers of the hippocampal formation, especially the dentate gyrus. The area postrema and intercolumnar tubercle contain moderate amounts. In the basal ganglia, brain stem and spinal cord, large neurons are found which contain abundant glycogen. Extracerebral blood vessel walls also contain some of the polysaccharide.

White matter ordinarily shows no glycogen. However, recent biochemical results obtained by Folbergrová et al. (1970) show that cerebral white matter of mouse brain contains about 30% more glycogen and glucose than does the cerebral cortex! Also, Mori and Leblond (1969) have recently shown by electron microscopy studies that glycogen is normally seen in fibrous astrocytes of the rat corpus callosum.

Cytologically, apart from the large neurons mentioned above, glycogen granules are localizable, but with difficulty, in neuronal perikarya; the task is made easier by using perfusion fixation (Shimizu and Kumamoto, 1952) and electron microscopy. While Koizumi and Shiraishi (1970) could not find glycogen in the perikarya of rabbit hypothalamic and cerebellar cortical neurons they did see some in some pre- and postsynaptic sites; this confirmed light microscopic observations by Shimizu and Kumamoto (1952) and others. On the other hand both by light and electron microscopy glycogen granules were frequently seen in astrocytic perikarya, as well as processes, especially the perivascular end-feet. Granules in "neuropil" seen by light microscopy must then be ascribed to those present in structurally unrecognizable neuroglial and/or neuronal processes.

It should be added here that some prominent species differences are seen. Among the rodents for example, it is the neurons of the basal amygdaloid, septal, hypoglossal, inferior olivary, trigeminal, mesencephalic, lateral reticular and ventral horn nuclei of the rat that contain most glycogen, while in the rabbit glycogen occurs mainly in the lateral hypothalamic, subthalamic, hypoglossal and spinal cord ventral horn nuclei as well as in the globus pallidus, zona incerta, nucleus ambiguous and tuber cinerum (Koizumi and Shiraishi, 1970).

The reason(s) for this seeming species difference, and the disparity between biochemical and histochemical results and between light and electron microscopic data, could, as mentioned above, be due to one or more of the following factors:

1. Varied regional rates of glycogenolysis dependent upon blood supply.

2. The physical state of the glycogen, determining as it does the rate with which it will be lysed, could be such that it allows easy loss of the glycogen from some sites more than others.

3. The physical state of the glycogen could allow its selective loss through simple differential solubility (see above).

4. The glycogen could be in a form that eludes histochemical detection, e.g. a form too dispersed to permit visibility in granular form (see Guth and Watson, 1968).

3. Phosphorylase (and Branching Enzyme)

3.1. Biochemical Considerations

In this summary* the enzymes phosphorylase and branching enzyme of various sources will be discussed together and data peculiar to CNS will be pointed out when necessary.

Phosphorylase belongs to one of two enzyme systems capable of the *in vitro* synthesis of α-1$\rightarrow$4-linkages of glycogen, the other being glycogen synthetase; branching enzyme is responsible for the periodic synthesis of the α-1$\rightarrow$6-linkages (see above). Phosphorylase catalyzes this reversibly (Cori and Cori, 1943) but, *in vivo*, it operates, together with a debranching enzyme, towards glycogenolysis because of the high inorganic phosphate concentration relative to that of glucose-1-phosphate. It is an "SH-enzyme" which exists in 2 forms, an active "a" and an inactive "b" form. Phosphorylase "a" of muscle is made up of 4 identical subunits (monomers) each composed of: one polypeptide chain; one pyridoxal-5'-phosphate attached to it; another polypeptide chain (identical in all subunits) with one phosphate group bound to it; and one adenosine-5'-phosphate (AMP). The molecular weight of each subunit is about 125000 so that the molecular weight of phosphorylase "a" is about 500000 and the enzyme is regarded as a tetramer. Phosphorylase "b" is the dimer form with a molecular weight 250000; Villar-Palasi and Larner (1970) quote a figure of 185000 for phosphorylase "b" and 370000 for phosphorylase "a". Transformation of phosphorylase "b" $\rightarrow$ "a" and "a" $\rightarrow$ "b" takes place. The "b" $\rightarrow$ "a" involves tetramerization and the

* Based on articles by: Breckenridge and Crawford (1961), Krebs and Fischer (1962, 1964), Breckenridge and Norman (1962, 1965), Fischer, Appleman and Krebs (1964), Krebs, Love, Bratvold, Trayser, Meyer and Fischer (1964), Fischer, Hurd, Koh, Seery and Teller (1968), Larner, Villar-Palasi, Goldberg, Bishop, Huijing, Wenger, Sasko and Brown (1968), Breckenridge and Johnston (1969), Villar-Palasi and Larner (1970), Shimizu, Tanaka, Suzuki and Matsukado (1971), Palmer, Schmidt and Robison (1972), Sutherland (1972) and Watanabe and Passonneau (1973).

transfer of 4 phosphate groupings from ATP ($+ Mg^{2+}$); this transfer is assumed to unmask new sites of interaction enabling tetramerization to take place (Fischer et al., 1964). In "a" → "b" transformation the reverse takes place.

Activity of phosphorylase of *muscle*, and presumably that of CNS * (Breckenridge and Norman, 1962, 1965) is generally dependent on 3 parameters:

1. Monomer ⇔ dimer (phosphorylase "b") ⇔ tetramer (phosphorylase "a") transformations.

2. Presence of pyridoxal-5'-phosphate as cofactor.

3. Presence of AMP which actually binds itself to the enzyme, 1 mole per mole of enzyme monomer (see above); ATP can compete for this site with AMP but is ineffective as an activator (see below). This nucleotide, AMP, is essential for activity of the "b" from of the enzyme, which is about 2% active without it and 60–70% active with it, and increases the activity of the "a" form by a further 30–40%; it does this by making the enzymes more efficient catalysts, and, by inhibiting the action of phosphorylase phosphatase (Fig. 1). In CNS, normally the "a" form (activity without AMP) constitutes only about 13% of total phosphorylase (activity with AMP), i.e. most phosphorylase (87%) is, *in vivo*, as it is in muscle (see Sutherland and Rall, 1960), in the inactive "b" form (Breckenridge and Norman, 1965); more recently, Edwards, *et al.* (1974) quote a figure of 16% for the normal *in vivo* proportion of phosphorylase "a" in chick brain. This could be because phosphorylase "a" in the normal tissues, which are rich in glucose, may be in a form (T-form) that has a low avidity for AMP; significantly, in the presence of increased glycogen content the enzyme aquires a strong avidity for AMP (R-form of the enzyme) (Helmreich *et al.*, 1967) and would thus become activated.

The proportion of the two forms "a" and "b" could be changed by competition with AMP, not only by ATP (see above), but also by UDPG (Breckenridge and Norman, 1962) and glucose-6-phosphate (G-6-P) (Fischer *et al.*, 1968). Furthermore, certain factors, such as hypothermia, inhibit active phosphorylase, while others such as insulin, caffeine, cocaine, amphetamine, anoxia and ischaemia, stimulate it (Breckenridge and Norman, 1965). Anoxia and ischaemia do that, in fact, in a matter of seconds. Within 15–20 sec of postmortem anoxia active phosphorylase rises from 13% to about 60–75%; longer exposures diminish it again so that it drops to 25–30% by 3 min (Breckenridge and Norman, 1962, 1965). The probable mechanism of this will be discussed presently.

Liver phosphorylase "b" is similar to that of muscle in being a dimer. However, in the presence of AMP its activity rises from 2–3% to only 10–15%. As in CNS, its transformation into the active form involves its phosphorylation, but not tetramerization (Sutherland and Wosilait, 1956; Sutherland and Rall, 1960; Grillo, 1961; Krebs and Fischer, 1962, 1964). This active form is still only 70–85% as active as total phosphorylase and needs AMP to become 100% active.

The balance between phosphorylases "a" and "b" is maintained by a number of factors acting on 4 enzymes (Fig. 1). A phosphorylase b kinase (E.C. 2.7.1.38), in the presence of ATP, Mg^{2+} and cAMP, transforms the "b" to "a" form by phosphorylating and tetramerizing it in the case of muscle (and CNS) and by phosphorylating it only in the case of liver. This kinase is activated by the cAMP,

---

* Muscle and CNS phosphorylases are not immunologically identical but are closer to each other than to that of liver (Henion and Sutherland, 1957).

which transforms it from an inactive to an active form by stimulating a specific phosphorylase kinase; it is inhibited by ethylene diamine tetracetate (EDTA). A phosphorylase phosphatase (E.C. 3.1.3.17) transforms the "a" to the "b" form by removal of 4 phosphate groups from the "a" form and, in so doing, depolymerizing it to the dimer form in case of muscle, and by removal of 2 phosphate groups only in the case of liver; it is inhibited by AMP and fluoride ions. The cAMP is, in turn, under control of a synthesizing (cyclising) adenyl cyclase system which acts on ATP as substrate, and a hydrolytic (decyclising) phosphodiesterase (cyclic 3′,5′-nucleotide phosphodiesterase, E.C. 3.1.4.C).

Adenyl cyclase, which in brain is present in the highest concentration of the body (22 times as much as liver when the content in the latter is taken as unity; Robison et al., 1970), is under control of, and is affected by, several factors:

1. Depolarizing agents such as K^+ and electrical stimulation.

2. Biogenic amines (adrenaline, noradrenaline, histamine, 5-hydroxytryptamine (5-HT) and substances that increase them, e.g. amphetamine.

3. Adenosine and other related nucleotides—possibly as a compartmentalized pool—(Huang et al., 1971).

4. Adrenocorticotrophic hormone (ACTH), glucagon and fluoride ions.

5. Anoxia and ischaemia.

All of these factors stimulate its activity, which is measurable in terms of increased content of cAMP (Sutherland and Rall, 1960; Kakiuchi and Rall, 1968a, b; Breckenridge and Johnston, 1969; Palmer et al., 1969; Rall and Sattin, 1970; Robison et al., 1970; Shimizu et al., 1970; Huang et al., 1971; Schultz and Daly, 1973; Skolnick et al., 1973; Ewards et al., 1974). It should be mentioned, however, that Palmer et al and Edwards et al. do not include 5-HT and Edwards et al. exclude also noradrenaline, while Rall and Sattin believe that the elevation of cAMP by electrical stimulation and elevated K^+ is not due to direct action on adenyl cyclase. All of these factors act within seconds, e.g. decapitation (ischaemia) of rabbit causes an 8 fold increase of brain cAMP by 90 sec. This, of course in turn, could account for the rapid increase of active phosphorylase mentioned above, but according to Kakiuchi and Rall (1968b) increasing cAMP in vitro did not change the phosphorylase "a" content. However, in view of the in vitro nature of the study, their finding can not be taken as conclusive; this is supported by the combined in vivo and in vitro studies of Edwards et al. (1974).

The phosphodiesterase content of brain is 100 fold larger than that of adenyl cyclase. Nevertheless, these two enzymes must be either under different control mechanisms or are located differently for, as mentioned above, many factors can cause a very rapid increase in cAMP even as the phosphodiesterase is out of all proportion to adenyl cyclase. It is possible that during synthesis of cAMP conditions do not favour its breakdown since phosphodiesterase is inhibited by ATP and inorganic phosphate which are both substrate and product, respectively, of cAMP synthesis. Also, subcellular fractionation shows that the two enzymes are physically separated. Kakiuchi and Rall (1968a), Breckenridge and Johnston (1969), Cheung (1970) and Schmidt et al. (1971).

Phosphodiesterase may be stimulated by insulin, hence the depleting effect of insulin on cAMP (Cheung, 1970); this should contrast with the stimulatory effect of insulin on the activity of active phosphorylase mentioned above. Phosphodiesterase is inhibited by methylxanthines (theophylline and caffeine) and by papaverine, hence the central stimulatory action of these drugs as cAMP increases, and hence the increases in active phosphorylase by these drugs (Kakiuchi and Rall, 1968a; Cheung, 1970; Goldberg *et al.*, 1970).

3.2. Histochemical Demonstration *

Many different techniques have been employed in the histochemical localization of phosphorylase, active alone and total; activity of the branching enzyme together with that of total phosphorylase has also been studied. Table 1 includes most of the incubation media used and gives some of the findings obtained through their use in the CNS. All naturally employ large amounts of the substrate glucose-1-phosphate to push the phosphorylase activity towards glycogenesis instead of glycogenolysis. Otherwise many differences appear.

Tissue Preparation

The majority of studies have been done using fresh unfixed cryostat sections. Although fixation—using say cold acetone (Takeuchi and Glenner, 1961)—is unnecessary and will diminish enzymic activity minimally if kept brief, we (Ibrahim and Castellani, 1968) found that a 5 min. fixation (on rat CNS) obviously improved localization and eliminated some iodine-stainable artifacts. Godlewski (1963) had also shown previously that a 15 min fixation (on liver) stabilized phosphorylase "a".

In our histochemical studies (Ibrahim and Castellani) we stressed that material should be obtained as quickly after death as possible because of the already mentioned marked sensitivity of phosphorylase to anoxia. In one study Ibrahim (1968) could verify this histochemically by comparing brain quenched almost while the animal was alive with brains allowed to undergo postmortem change for variable lengths of time; however, the technique he employed is not practical or necessary for routine use. He also found that total phosphorylase began to diminish after about 5 min of anoxia (death). The conclusions of practical significance from these two studies were: 1. that brain tissue should be frozen within about 2 min of death for more accurate studies of total phosphorylase, with or without branching enzyme, 2. that histochemical demonstration of active phosphorylase alone does not represent the *in vivo* state, 3. that control material is essential, preferably from animals of the same age handled identically and simultaneously, and 4. that control, as well experimental material, should be placed on the same holder and cut in such a way as to counteract possible variations in thickness between them as this causes false results; cutting should be at 16–20 μm to allow proper cellular identification and optimal enzymic demonstration.

The volume of incubation medium as originally described is very large and, because of the expense involved, wasteful. We, therefore, employed a small uniform chambre technique in which sections on one or two slides (one inverted over the other) were incubated in about 0.6 ml; similar devises have been employed by others (e.g. Korsgaard and Wulff, 1967). The uniformity of the height of the chambre is essential since variations of this can lead to false results especi-

---

* For history and other aspects of the subject see Pearse (1972, p. 826).

Table 1. Techniques used to demonstrate phosphorylase or phosphorylase + branching enzymic activity[a]

Author	Incubation medium and tissue(s) studied	Findings in CNS
Yin and Sun (1947)	G-1-P, buffer[b] (soybeans, geranium leaves)	(P+B) Not reported
Goldberg et al. (1952)	G-1-P, fluoride, buffer (liver, kidney, uterus)	(P+B) Not reported
Cobb (1949), Cobb and Lafayette (1953)	G-1-P, barium chloride, buffer (cartilage, developing bone)[c]	(P+B) Not reported
Takeuchi and Kuriaki (1955)	G-1-P, G, AMP, insulin, buffer (brain, liver, muscles, cartilage)	(P+B) No activity (none reported in liver either)
Takeuchi et al. (1955)	G-1-P, G, AMP, insulin, buffer (as Takeuchi, 1958)	(P+B) Activity confined to blood vessels and grey matter
Shimizu and Okada (1957)	G-1-P, AMP, insulin (brain)	(P+B) Detailed topography but little cytology given; white matter and many grey areas[+++]
Takeuchi (1958)	G-1-P, G, AMP, insulin, buffer, ethanol, (CNS, liver, skeletal muscle, skeleton visceral organs)	(P) Grey matter stronger than white; large neurons of spinal cord[+++]
Takeuchi (1956, 1965a)	G-1-P, G, AMP, insulin, buffer, ethanol (Purkinje fibers, brain)	(P) Neuronal perikarya, axons and neuroglia[++]
Friede (1959a, b, 1966)[d]	G-1-P, G, ATP, monoiodoacetate (brain)	(P+B) White matter stronger than grey, mainly axonal, rare in glia; Purkinje cells and Bergmann glia[+++]
Grillo (1961)	G-1-P, G, AMP (or cyclic-AMP), Mg, adrenaline (or glucagon), buffer, ethanol (muscle, liver, cartilage)	(P) Not reported
Hess and Pearse (1961)	Same as Takeuchi (1956, 1958) (skeletal muscle)	(P) Not reported
Eränkö and Palkama (1961)	G-1-P, G, AMP, insulin, buffer, ethanol, fluoride, PVP (muscle and liver)	(P) Not reported
Guha and Wegmann (1961)	G-1-P, ATP-Mg, AMP (or cyclic-AMP), fluoride, adrenaline (liver of chick embryo)	(P+B) Not reported
Wegmann and Sotelo (1963)	As Guha and Wegmann (1961) (sciatic nerve)	(P+B) Axoplasm[+++], Nodes of Ranvier[++]
Sasaki and Takeuchi (1963)	G-1-P, G, AMP, insulin, buffer, ethanol, sucrose (skeletal muscle)	(P) Not reported
Godlewksi (1963)	G-1-P, ATP-Mg, AMP, fluoride, EDTA (arterial wall)	(P+B) Not reported
Sotelo and Wegmann (1964)	On blocks (as Friede 1959) or sections (as Guha and Wegmann, 1961) (cerebellum)	(P+B) Fibrous astrocytes[+++] oligodendrocytes[++], nerve fibers[+], Purkinje cell dendrites[+]
Takeuchi (1965b)	G-1-P, G, AMP (or ATP-Mg or glucagon), fluoride (brain)	(P+B) Activity in neuronal perikarya and axons
Bo and Smith (1965)	G-1-P, G, AMP, insulin, buffer, ethanol (smooth muscle)	(P) Not reported

Table 1 (continued)

Author	Incubation medium and tissue(s) studied	Findings in CNS	
Guha and Wegmann (1965, 1966)	Same as (1961), ^{14}C-G-1-P and autoradiography (muscle, liver, rectum, skin)	(P+B)	Not reported
Hori (1966a)[e]	G-1-P, AMP, buffer, fluoride, EDTA (liver)	(P+B)	Not reported
Mossakowski et al. (1967)	G-1-P, AMP, ATP-Mg, fluoride, EDTA (developing brain)	(P+B)	White or grey matter neuropil + or ++, with few exceptions neurons, neuroglia and vessels—no activity
Korsgaard and Wulff (1967)	G-1-P, G, AMP, buffer, fluoride, PVP (liver, muscle, skin, rectal mucosa)	(P+B)	Not reported
Meijer (1968a, b)	G-1-P, AMP, buffer, fluoride, dextran, EDTA (liver, muscles)	(P+B)	Not reported
Ibrahim and Castellani (1968) and Ibrahim et al. (1970a, b)	G-1-P, G, AMP, insulin, buffer, ethanol, fluoride, PVP (CNS)	(P)	Neuronal perikarya, axons, neuropil, astrocytes, oligodendroglia and vessels +++
Lindberg and Palkama (1972)	G-1-P, insulin, buffer, ethanol, fluoride, PVP, EDTA (liver)	(P)	Not reported
Ibrahim et al. (1973)	On blocks or fresh frozen sections as Eränkö and Palkama, 1961 (brain)	(P+B) and (P)	Complementary picture demonstrating all elements

[a] Modified from Ibrahim et al. (1973).
[b] Buffer between pH 5.7 and 6.0 and incubation usually at 37° C.
[c] Frozen-dried material embedded in carnauba wax.
[d] Fresh thick blocks incubated and then embedded in paraffin.
[e] Fresh frozen and freeze-substituted material; all other material was fresh frozen.
G = Glycogen; (P) = Phosphorylase demonstrated; (P+B) = Phosphorylase + branching enzyme demonstrated. + = weak, ++ = moderate, +++ = strong activity.

ally if a section is large or if control and experimental material are side by side (see Fig. 5b and Ibrahim and Castellani, 1968).

Apart from the widespread use of frozen sections a few studies by Friede (1959a, b), Sotelo and Wegmann (1964) and Ibrahim, Pascoe and Khayat (1973) were done on thick blocks of tissue (1–2 mm) which were incubated as such and then embedded in paraffin. The results of these were somewhat different from those using cryostat sections but both tended to complement each other (see p. 29).

The Incubation Media

These have varied depending on the theoretical views of the workers using them (see Table 1).

The Use of a Primer

Use of glycogen as a primer is established biochemically, but histochemically it has been advocated by some and not by others. Although Ibrahim and Castellani (1968) found that glycogen primer was not essential for phosphorylase activity, *full* activity was not possible without it; this supported previous conclusions of Takeuchi and co-workers (1955), Eränkö and Palkama (1961), Hess and Pearse (1961) and Bo and Smith (1965). It is significant that the majority of workers who did not use a primer used tissues usually replete with intrinsic glycogen, e.g. muscle and liver. Such glycogen could act as a nucleus on which further glucoses attach; the amount of glycogen which goes into solution from rich sites into the incubation medium (Hori, 1966a) could also act as a primer for poor sites. Nervous tissue, being relatively poor in glycogen, should then need extrinsic (added) primer (Ibrahim and Castellani, 1968). The findings of Meijer (1968a, b), based on combined biochemical and histochemical studies of normal liver and skeletal muscle, and, more significantly on anoxic and ischaemic dog heart, tend to show that extraneous glycogen primer is useless. This is supposedly because of the high molecular weight of commercially available soluble glycogens ($2.5-5 \times 10^6$) which probably prevents their penetration into cells. It should be remembered, however, that plasma membranes of cells in tissue cryostat sections do not behave as they would *in vivo* and besides, intrinsic glycogen molecules of even higher molecular weight (see Glycogen) do leave the cells in the opposite direction to dissolve in incubation media. It is also possible that tissue phosphorylase and debranching enzyme, as well as amylases (see below), partially break down extrinsic glycogen to smaller more suitable forms.

Meijer's use of dextrans of molecular weight 19900–2000000 proved quite useful in his hands especially in areas of anoxic or ischaemic cardiac muscle. This muscle had been depleted completely of glycogen and showed no histochemically demonstrable, but still biochemically surviving, phosphorylase activity. Under these conditions he found that, "it is essential to use as acceptor an unbranched dextran fraction with a high average molecular weight" (200000 to 2000000). This he concluded is because as the molecular weight of the dextran rises so does the affinity of phosphorylase for it; this same relationship has already been shown for the affinity of glycogen to phosphorylase (Tata, 1964). It should be mentioned that Lindberg and Palkama (1972) found that neither glycogen nor dextran enhanced phosphorylase activity. However, Meijer used liver and muscle and Lindberg and Palkama used liver which are known to have high intrinsic glycogen.

The Use of Activators and Inhibitors

Workers in the field have studied different tissues (liver, muscle, CNS, etc.) and have based their techniques and the composition of their media on the known biochemical data concerning each tissue. Thus for instance, as mentioned under "Biochemical Considerations", full activation of phosphorylase can logically be achieved in several ways, apart from the traditional use of promptly frozen tissue, high G-1-P levels and optimal pH and temperature of incubation:

1. *Nucleotides.* These have included AMP, ATP and cAMP. AMP is a logical choice since it activates phosphorylase "b" of muscle and CNS (not of liver significantly), activates phosphorylase "a" fully and inhibits phosphorylase phosphatase. Therefore, its inclusion gives the full or total phosphorylase activity. ATP should have a two-sided effect. On the one hand it can be harmful since it can compete with the activator AMP (see above and also Kahn and Blum, 1971), but on the other hand it can provide the necessary phosphate groupings to transform phosphorylase "b" to "a", and is the substrate for adenyl cyclase which

transforms it to cAMP; it also inhibits phosphodiesterase which hydrolyses the cAMP, and therefore helps maintain the level of the latter, once it is formed. cAMP, in turn, is useful since it activates phosphorylase b kinase which transforms phosphorylase "b" to "a" (see p. 13).

Therefore, we see that for tissues, other than liver, inclusion of AMP should, *per se*, be a sufficiently good activation to demonstrate total phosphorylase activity. The use of ATP or cAMP, without added AMP, should not be as efficient since even the AMP, released as the end-product of the hydrolysis of ATP, would not be sufficient or available fast enough to activate the phosphorylases. In fact, Hess and Pearse (1961) have shown for skeletal muscle that "the phosphorylase reaction was inhibited by substituiting ---------------------- (ATP), --------------------- (ADP), or cyclic adenosine-3',5'-phosphate for ---------------------- (AMP) in the medium". Also Ibrahim and Castellani found that with AMP, cAMP, ATP ($+ Mg^{2+}$), ADP and no nucleotide, demonstrable activity of phosphorylase in brain was less and less in that order.

On the other hand, for liver it is logical to have ATP ($+ Mg^{2+}$), AMP and cAMP all at the same time since phosphorylase "b"—normally only 10–15% active even in the presence of AMP (see above)—has first to be transformed to the "a" type (through $ATP + Mg^{2+}$ and cAMP). This, together with the phosphorylase "a" already present, still needs AMP for its full activation (see p. 13).

2. *Adrenaline and Glucagon*. These two hormones activate adenyl cyclase and hence theoretically could be given, especially in the case of liver, to stimulate the necessary step of cAMP formation.

3. *Insulin*. As mentioned above this stimulates active phosphorylase, and its use is therefore logical and widespread; it must be assumed that its stimulatory effect on phosphodiesterase (Cheung, 1970), and hence tendency to lower levels of cAMP, must be adequately counterbalanced.

4. *Fluoride*. This also is a logical choice, first made by Goldberg et al. (1952), since it inhibits phosphorylase phosphatase (and nonspecific phosphatase) and hence prevents phosphorylase "a" to "b" transformation. It also stimulates adenyl cyclase with its consequent activating effects. Furthermore, it inhibits transformation of G-1-P to G-6-P by phosphoglucomutase by inhibiting this enzyme; G-6-P formed in this way means lost G-1-P (Hori, 1964, 1966b).

5. *EDTA*. First used by Godlewski, this chelating agent has been used by several workers since. Until the time of Hori (1966a) it was known that EDTA inhibited phosphorylase b kinase thus preventing phosphorylase "b" to "a" conversion. This, in itself, was no advantage except when activity of *phosphorylase "a" alone* was sought (see Godlewski, 1963). However, EDTA was also found to have a stimulatory effect on phosphorylase increasing the polyglucose yield of incubation. This, according to Hori (1966a), could be due to (i) prevention of the enzyme or the polyglucose from going into solution in the medium, (ii) protection of intrinsic glycogen and polyglucose from α-amylase, (iii) protection of phosphorylase "a" from inactivation by salts and ions, (iv) direct stimulation of phosphorylase "a" and/or (v) activation of the branching enzyme. Hori had used liver for his studies, had not used a primer (extrinsic glycogen) and had found that EDTA caused 40–50% of intrinsic glycogen of sections to be retained there. This, obviously therefore, provided the necessary primer and in such unusually large amounts and in a natural form so that the increased polyglucose yield could be attributed, at least partly, to this; one or more of the other possible

mechanisms listed by Hori could be operative also. Lindberg and Palkama (1972), who advocate the use of EDTA because it improved activity of phosphorylase (in liver), do not really know how it accomplishes this. It is pertinent perhaps that Kahn and Blum (1971) found that phosphorylase of Tetrahymena pyriformis was, in fact, inhibited, and irreversibly, by EDTA. In view of the inadequate information on the exact mode of action of EDTA, some controversies, and the real danger of interference of too much retained intrinsic glycogen with the final picture, we, as well as others (Table 1), have avoided its use for demonstration of total phosphorylase and phosphorylase + branching enzyme. However, its use is obviously essential for demonstration of active phosphorylase alone, provided it is remembered that by routine techniques this does not really represent the *in vivo* state.

6. *Monoiodoacetate*. This was used only by Friede (1959 a, b) who found that it improved the reaction on *en block* incubation. This may be attributed to its blockage of glycolysis, being an SH-inhibitor. The use of this compound has apparently not been considered for thin section work; because of its SH inhibition it must necessarily diminish phosphorylase activity.

7. *Ethanol*. The addition of this alcohol to the original medium of Takeuchi and Kuriaki (1955) by Takeuchi (1958 and references there) was not to limit diffusion of the polyglucose product (Korsgaard and Wulff, 1967). It was based on knowledge from biochemical data that ethanol (and $HgCl_2$) inhibit the branching enzyme which, if not thus suppressed, would take part in the synthesis of the polyglucose causing its branching (Takeuchi, 1958; Meijer, 1968a). Ethanol does, however, also accelerate precipitation of the newly-formed polyglucose (Takeuchi, 1958).

As might be expected, the medium devoid of a branching enzyme inhibitor (e.g. ethanol) was shown to produce an "amyolpectin- or glycogen-type" polyglucose, while a medium that included ethanol produced a straight chain amylose-type (see above); the manner in which the new chains are added on to an original "nucleus-primer" must be very similar to that described below for glycogen synthetase by Manners (1968). When stained with iodine, the branched polyglucose gave a violet or brownish purple colour, and was completely digestible with α-amylase but incompletely digestible with β-amylase. On the other hand, the amylose gave a blue colour and was completely digestible with both α- and β-amylases. Therefore, a section, incubated in a medium devoid of ethanol and then digested with β-amylase and stained with iodine, demonstrates activity of phosphorylase + branching enzyme, not just of branching enzyme as is sometimes loosely said. However, comparison of two media ± ethanol, digested as directed, should indicate the state of activity of branching enzyme. It should be added that incubation in a medium devoid of ethanol, and staining with iodine, shows a whole range of colours including all the above plus, sometimes, a red-brown or mahogany colour of original unextracted glycogen. These colours, especially in suitably-digested sections, do then reflect the state of complexity of the polyglucose of incubation (Swanson, 1948; Takeuchi et al., 1955; Takeuchi, 1958; Sasaki and Takeuchi, 1963; Takeuchi and Sasaki, 1970; Ibrahim et al., 1973).

Takeuchi et al. had drawn attention to the slightly inhibiting effect of ethanol (20%) on phosphorylase activity, as have Korsgaard and Wulff (1967) more recently. The latter authors, losing sight of the original reason behind the use of ethanol, understandably found it not only unnecessary but harmful; this applies to all authors who do not use ethanol in their incubation medium and who are supposed to be demonstrating phosphorylase but are in fact demonstrating phosphorylase + branching enzyme.

It should be mentioned as well that ethanol, like fluoride, inhibits phosphoglucomatase which is another advantage to its use (see above).

8. *Polyvinyl pyrrolidone (PVP)*. Apart from the coincidental effect of ethanol in the partial limitation of diffusion of synthesized polyglucose, another technique, employed first by Eränkö and Palkama (1961), was the use of PVP at a concentration of 7.5%. Because of the high molecular weight of PVP (appx. 24000) these authors believed that it functioned because of the increase in viscosity rather than because of an osmotic effect. The use of PVP has been advocated by several authors since (Table 1), and has proved invaluable. Korsgaard and Wulff (1967) used an even higher concentration (200 mg/ml) of a PVP (m.w. = 12000). They found that such an increase in viscosity enhanced reaction in all tissues studied (liver, skin, striated muscle and colonic epithelium). They could also use thinner sections than usually recommended (8–10 μm instead of 16–40 μm) and the sections were well protected. Diffusion of the soluble phosphorylase enzyme was also said to be limited by the use of PVP.

With all the above considerations it is apparent then that, on the whole, the medium of Eränkö and Palkama, which of course is based on that used by Takeuchi *et al.*, is the best choice especially for use on CNS material; addition of more PVP, as advocated by Korsgaard and Wulff could be useful. We have used stock solutions of this medium (500 ml) containing all ingredients except ethanol and kept in cold storage (4°C) for months without obvious deterioration. For use, the medium was allowed to reach room temperature, shaken vigorously and filtered directly onto the sections if activity of phosphorylase + branching enzyme was required. For total phosphorylase alone ethanol was added, 0.5 ml to 2.5 ml of stock solution, just before use; the same stock solution devoid of AMP was used for active phosphorylase and to it ethanol and EDTA were added as above. The reason for shaking was to redissolve the glycogen primer some of which precipitated out in the cold.

The incubation time we found varied according to the tissue tested and the enzymic activity sought. Thus, in the case of CNS, incubation for phosphorylase alone required 2 hr; phosphorylase + branching enzyme required $^1/_2$ hr only. This we attributed to the absence of ethanol, which as mentioned inhibits phosphorylase a little, and may be also to the newly synthesized branched polyglucose which could start chain-reaction formation of more polyglucose by providing more and more suitable nidation centers. Even shorter incubation time was necessary for skeletal muscle and liver; phosphorylase alone $^1/_2$–1 hr, phosphorylase + branching $^1/_4$–$^1/_2$ hr.

Procedure after Incubation

The products of enzymic activity are two, polyglucoses of varying chain length and side branching, and phosphate moieties. Both of these can be demonstrated.

1. *Polyglucose*. Wheather this is amylose-, amylopectin- or glycogen-like it is soluble in water to varying degrees. Therefore, incubated sections could be shaken of excess medium and, with or without prior fixation in absolute ethanol, plunged

directly into dilute Gram's iodine (see Glycogen) or stained in some other way (see p. 10). Or, they could be washed briefly in 40% ethanol and then, with or without prior drying, fixed in absolute ethanol, air dried and then stained. This we found was the method of choice and is recommended.

For visualization of the polyglucose there are three approaches. The first of these involves its staining and the method of choice is still, as just mentioned, staining with dilute Gram's iodine (see Yin and Sun, 1947). This has the big advantage of being the only way of obtaining a visual impression of the chain length and branching of the polyglucose(s) end-product, especially when branching enzyme is included; surviving intrinsic glycogen is also stained differently. The main drawback is the eventual fading of the iodine colour, especially in the light. This, however, can be counteracted by storage in the dark and cold and by prompt studying and photography if needed. These sections could then be destained with absolute ethanol and restained with the permanent PAS procedure. An alternative is to restain faded sections (usually mounted in iodine-glycerine) in dilute Gram's iodine; such staining differs in no way from the original. Another alternative is to use initially one of the recommended techniques advocated for "permanent" iodine staining (Takeuchi and Kuriaki, 1955; Smith et al., 1966; Sawyer et al., 1965). We tried such "permanent" staining but found it altered original colours such that the value of iodine staining no longer held. Also, with long storage, fading still occurred, only then cover slips could not be easily removed and the slides restained.

The other method of staining the polyglucose is by the PAS technique which has been in use since Goldberg et al. (1952) and Cobb and Lafayette (1953). This, when combined with aldehyde blockade (Bulmer, 1959), staines, more or less specifically, glycogen and other polyglucoses (Guha and Wegmann, 1966; Ibrahim et al., 1970b). Its advantage is permanency but its disadvantage is the lack of varied shades of colour of iodine staining with their significance (see also Takeuchi and Sasaki, 1970). Used after destaining of iodine-stained preparations it is very useful; alcoholic-PAS gave us better results than the usual PAS (Ibrahim and Castellani, 1968).

The third method of staining is by Best's carmine, first employed by Goldberg et al. and later by Takeuchi and Kuriaki (1955). As with the PAS technique it stains both glycogen and glycogen-like polyglucoses similarly. This, coupled with its greater technical difficulty, makes its use limited.

The second approach is the use of autoradiography. Guha and Wegmann (1965, 1966) devised such a technique in which they used C^{14}-G-1-P as substrate (Table 1). Parallel sections stained traditionally confirmed the presence of radioactivity at sites of PAS- and iodine-stainable polyglucose. The main advantages of this techniques are twofold: (i) It demonstrates conclusively the new synthesis of polyglucose and its location without confusion from any unextracted glycogen. (ii) It can demonstrate sites of low phosphorylase activity which could "escape detection by the iodine method because the chain length of the glycogen synthesized is too short to be coloured by iodine" (Guha and Wegmann, 1965).

The third approach is by visualizing the polyglucose by electron microscopy. Neosynthesis of polyglucose has been demontrated in this way after histochemical incubation by Sasaki and Takeuchi (1963) and Takeuchi and Sasaki (1970). Obvious morphological differences were noted in skeletal muscle between native glycogen and newly-synthesized polyglucose which, in itself, also varied depending upon wheather polyglucose was synthesized through phosphorylase or glycogen synthetase. Such differences were reflected in variations in molecular weight and tinctorial characteristics with iodine staining. These authors also noted that in skeletal muscle smooth endoplasmic reticulum is in close association with glycogen-rich areas and, therefore, may be involved in its synthesis and breakdown. They also concluded that phosphorylase and branching enzyme are "perhaps localized in the same area"; this has bearing on further discussion.

2. *Phosphate.* This has been visualized both at the light and the electron microscope levels. The significance of this approach has not been so much its routine applicability but rather its use for demonstrating phosphorylase activity ultrastructurally. First conceived by Goldberg *et al.* (1952), this technique was designed on the basis of the Gomori type of reaction for demonstrating phosphatases. It entails the inclusion of a lead salt in the incubation medium to capture the phosphate groupings as they are released. Subsequent demonstration of lead phosphate is by exposure to dilute yellow ammonium sulphide to form black lead sulphide.

Feasible in theory, this technique gave the same localization as when polyglucose was stained. However, Hori (1964) found the method was somewhat unreliable and modified it to give reproducible results in liver and muscle of rat. He also fixed the tissues in buffered 2.5% glutaraldehyde at 0°C for 2 hr and included fluoride and ethanol in his medium to obviate the possibility of non-specific phosphatase and phosphoglucomutase activity leading to false results (see above); artifactual localization due to a specific G-1-Pase is out of the question because there is no G-1-Pase in animal tissues. In muscle, localization of activity corresponded well to that of polyglucose. He employed as well lead nitrate at 3.6 mM concentration but in a later paper (Hori, 1966b) he used a 4.2 mM concentration and demonstrated the radioopaque lead by electron microscopy and lead sulphide by light microscopy. In liver there was, however, some discrepancy between location of lead sulphide and polyglucose. Ultrastructurally, he confirmed that the reaction product was in close association with endoplasmic reticulum.

Meijer (1968a) used the same principles when he showed that dextran can replace glycogen as primer (see above).

Later, Lindberg and Palkama (1970a, b) denied completely that demonstration of phosphorylase was possible by this technique since lead ions inhibit the enzyme. Nevertheless, in a subsequent communication (1972) they conceded that demonstration was possible provided lead concentration was kept low (0.4 mM). Their final recommendation was not, on the whole, favourable to the technique as such.

Criticism of the Takeuchi Techniques for Phosphorylase Demonstration

Recently, Eckner (1968, 1969), Eckner (1971) and Martin and Engel (1972) have shed doubts on the validity of the Takeuchi-type techniques employed for the visualization of phosphorylase activity. The criticisms of Eckner *et al.* are based on studies by Krug *et al.* (1967) which showed that in infarcted cardiac muscle only those fibers containing glycogen demonstrated phosphorylase activity. Eckner *et al.* (1969) followed this up by a study in normal freeze-dried cardiac muscle and liver of phosphorylase, phosphorylase + branching enzyme and glycogen synthetase activities. They found that sites devoid of demonstrable glycogen did not aquire any polyglucose after incubation for the enzymes, and if glycogen had been present, the amounts of final product after incubation were even less than what was initially present. This meant that neosynthesis of polyglucose through enzyme activity had not occurred and that some of the pre-existent glycogen had been dissolved out by the incubation medium. They incubated control sections in buffer without G-1-P (or UDPG) and found that some glycogen still remained. Their final conclusion was that the solubility and extraction of pre-existent glycogen could be inhibited by the various substrates in the incubation media; this they thought could explain the close correlation between glycogen, phosphorylase and glycogen synthetase. They further believed that it was possible that the enzymic reactions occurred in the incubating solution rather than in the tissue section and hence no synthesis of polysaccharide is localizable in sections.

There are several studies that can explain the findings of Krug *et al.* and refute the conclusions of the others. The first is a study in two parts by Meijer (1968a, b) directed at this very problem, which puzzled himself as well as others (see references in Meijer, 1968a), viz. "why the presence of phosphorylase activity in glycogen-depleted muscle fibres" could not be demonstrated histochemically while biochemical analysis showed its presence. He found that the explanation lay in the fact that once tissue glycogen is depleted, as by anoxia or ischaemia, no extrinsic glycogen could act as a primer. This he attributed to the high molecular weight of the glycogen used as an extrinsic primer. He therefore, used a dextran as the primer and found that then such muscle fibers did show synthesis of some polyglucose. This did not apply to severely damaged muscle, however, for any surviving phosphorylase in such muscle probably denatured too much.

The second study is by Cobb (1949) and Cobb and Lafayette (1953). They found that they could remove all glycogen from maturing bone and cartilage and yet retain demonstrable phosphorylase activity. However, Goldberg *et al.* (1952) found that removal of glycogen by the methods of Cobb and Cobb and Lafayette (use of saliva, diastase or just buffer) also removed all demontrable enzymic activity in *normal* liver, kidney and uterus.

The third study is by Ibrahim *et al.* (1973) which also attempted removal of glycogen with retention of phosphorylase. Cryostat sections of ischaemic-hypoxic rat brains (Levine, 1960) were treated as follows:

1. Some were fixed in ethanol for 2–4 hr, dried in air and stained with Gram's iodine or dimedone-PAS to show the glycogen distribution.

2. Some were incubated for phosphorylase activity for 2 hr and stained as above.

3. Some were extracted by incubation in the medium for phosphorylase without glycogen primer or G-1-P at 37°C for periods of up to 1 hr and then stained as above; Takeuchi and Sasaki (1970) had shown that 1 hr or longer, was needed to extract intrinsic glycogen from frozen sections incubated at room temperature.

4. Some were treated as in (3) and then incubated in the complete medium for phosphorylase for 2 hr and stained as usual.

Although not all glycogen was removed from the extracted sections the results showed that new polyglucose was synthesized. Furthermore, such sections did contain large areas in which no glycogen could be stained. These depleted areas had less but still obvious new polyglucose after incubation for total phosphorylase activity. This clearly showed that extraction of glycogen does not interfere with the demonstration of phosphorylase activity provided sufficient glycogen primer is present in the medium; the problem of the primer was discussed above. The incompleteness of extraction of pathologically-induced polyglucose (or glycogen?) from areas adjacent to necrotic ones must be attributed to unknown factors of molecular size and bond to tissue constituents altering its extractability (Smitherman et al., 1972).

Martin and Engel (1972) depleted cat gastrocnemius and soleus muscles of glycogen by exhaustion through prolonged electrical stimulation. Histochemically, phosphorylase activity in these muscles was greatly diminished but biochemically it was normal. Although made with some reservation, the conclusion of these authors was that the demonstration of phosphorylase histochemically depends upon sufficient quantities of intrinsic rather than extrinsic glycogen primer. This conclusion may seem to be valid but it should be pointed out that first of all these authors used the original unrefined medium of Takeuchi and Kuriaki (1955) to demonstrate phosphorylase activity; this medium does not fulfill several of the criteria mentioned above that are necessary for optimal demonstration of activity. Furthermore, it is probable that, as in the case of the starved liver (Tata, 1964; Sie et al., 1964), the enzyme is set free from the granular form of glycogen as this goes into the soluble phase of the cell (see p. 33); as mentioned above, glycogen exists reversibly in several forms including a soluble form (Smitherman et al., 1972). Moreover, Tata (1964) has shown that the larger the molecular weight of glycogen (large granular form) the more firmly it binds phosphorylase and presumably vice versa. If the enzyme is indeed set free in the tetanized muscle then enzymic diffusion has to be checked by addition of PVP before its activity can be demonstrated histochemically. Furthermore, it is possible that the enzyme might become more easily inactivated by phosphorylase phosphatase and hence the presence of fluoride ions in the medium becomes quite necessary. Such requirements are apparently unnecessary in biochemical assays of the enzyme whether it be particulate or soluble. It is perhaps significant that with adequate media, Fagundes and Cohen (1965) demonstrated histochemically increases in phosphorylase activity in liver lobules depleted of glycogen by starvation. We have made the same observation (unpublished observations).

The attempt by Martin and Engel to facilitate the reaction with unusually large amounts of extrinsic primer was self-defeating since high concentrations of glycogen would inhibit, rather than stimulate, phosphorylase activity (Takeuchi and Kuriaki, 1955).

When we repeated the histochemical portion of the experiment of Martin and Engel (Ibrahim et al., 1973), we found that the Takeuchi-Kuriaki medium (1955) gave poor results but no difference in enzyme activity between control and experimental muscles. Incubation in a combination of enriched media (Eränkö and Palkama, 1961; Lindberg and Plakama, 1972) gave much better results. In no case was diminution of phosphorylase activity visible (Ibrahim et al., in preparation). Therefore, at least in the more physiological exhausted muscle, incubation in adequate media showed that depletion of glycogen was not accompanied by a change in histochemical activity of phosphorylase; these results are in agreement with the biochemical analyses of phosphorylase by Martin and Engel. The situation regarding pathologically-induced changes in glycogen and its enzymes is probably different as will be pointed out later.

Further confirmation of the validity of the "Takeuchi techniques" is provided indirectly by the various iodine colour reactions of polyglucoses and by the demonstration of polyglucose neosynthesis by all the various techniques mentioned above (Goldberg *et al.*, 1952; Sasaki and Takeuchi, 1963; Guha and Wegmann, 1965; Hori, 1964, 1966a, b; Meijer, 1968a; Takeuchi and Sasaki, 1970; Lindberg and Palkama, 1972). It is of interest also that Wanson and Drochmans (1968) found that isolated glycogen particles, when incubated in a medium containing G-1-P, AMP and NaF at pH 6.1, grew in size aquiring on their surface new minute granules (40 Å) and filamentous forms of synthesized polyglucose.

In conclusion, therefore, we feel that criticisms of the validity of the techniques of Takeuchi *et al.* are unfounded.

3.3 Normal Distribution

Essentially, phosphorylase and phosphorylase + branching enzyme have the same distribution as glycogen, including in the retina (Hutchinson and Kuwabara, 1962; Niemi, 1965). However, there are some differences between them depending on the age of the animal studied, the location in the CNS, the degree of hypoxia (or anoxia) to which the tissue was exposed and wheather cryostat sections, or paraffin sections of brains incubated *en bloc*, were used to study the enzymes (Takeuchi, 1956, 1958, 1965a, b; Shimizu and Okada, 1957; Friede 1959a b, 1966; Sotelo and Wegmann, 1964; Eckner *et al.*, 1968, 1969; Ibrahim *et al.*, 1970a, 1973) (see Table 1). Thus for instance, newborn rats showed least enzymic activity which increased gradually over a few days to a maximum at 21 days of age (Shimizu and Okada, 1957). Again, although Ibrahim *et al.*, (1970a) found white matter showed practically no histochemically-demonstrable glycogen (see p. 11), yet its phosphorylase content was easily demonstrated, but differed thus: In cryostat sections, incubated for phosphorylase + branching enzyme and stained with iodine, choroid plexus (Fig. 2A), leptomeninges, axons, astrocytes and oligodendrocytes contained purplish deposits (Fig. 2B). On the other hand, in paraffin sections treated similarly only strongly active astrocytes and prominent 'beaded' axons were present within very pale 'neuropil' (Fig. 2D). Activity in grey matter areas also differed. In cryostat sections incubated for phosphorylase + branching enzyme fine brown or purple granules were numerous in the neuropil to the point of almost obscuring cellular identity (Fig. 2C). Nevertheless, a brownish colour was distinguishable in neuronal perikarya, and a purple colour in ill-defined neuroglia and 'neuropil' (Fig. 2C); the cerebral and cerebellar cortical molecular layers were especially dark (Fig. 2C) and large neurons of brainstem often showed strong purple activity. Paraffin sections differed in that most neurons of all sizes and some astrocytes were dark brown-purple and sharply outlined (Figs. 2E and F), while the 'neuropil' was generally pale but occasionally dark as in the cortical molecular layers (Fig. 2F). Sometimes, when neuronal perikarya were dark, astrocytes and 'neuropil' were light, and *vice versa*.

In the case of phosphorylase alone, cryostat sections of white matter showed more prominent astrocytes and oligodendrocytes staining bluish-green (Fig. 3B), while paraffin sections contained astrocytes only with a lightly granulated 'neuropil' (Fig. 3C). In grey matter, cryostat sections showed the same overall picture as seen with phosphorylase + branching enzyme except that the neuropil was

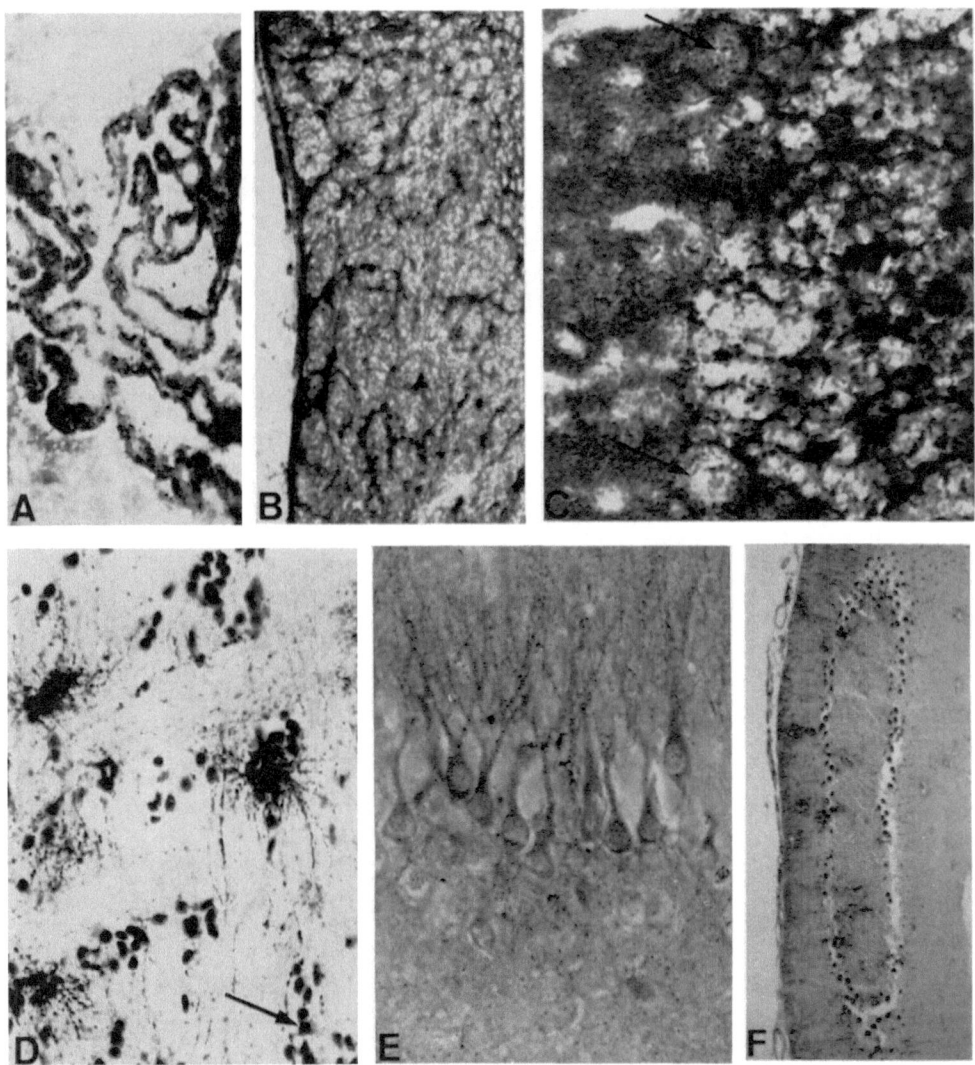

Fig. 2 A—F. Activity of phosphorylase + branching enzyme in normal rat brain. A, B and C are from cryostat sections and stained with dilute Gram's iodine. D, E and F are from paraffin sections and stained with Dimedone-PAS. (A) Choroid plexus. ×560. (B) Edge of pyramid in region of pons. Note leptomeninges, neuroglia (unidentifiable), axons and "neuropil". ×140. (C) Cerebellar cortex showing diffuse activity in molecular layer (left), particulate activity in flask-shaped Purkinje cells (arrows) and strong activity probably in granule cell perikarya, neuroglia and glomeruli of granule cell layer (right). Activity in Bergmann glia not prominent. ×560. (D) White matter (corpus callosum) with prominent activity in astrocytes and coursing axons. Little activity is localizable in probable oligodendroglia (arrow) and "neuropil". Counterstained with hematoxylin, ×370. (E) Pyramidal neurons of hippocampus, "neuropil" and adjacent molecular layers. ×350. (F) Cerebellar cortex, in which most prominent activity is in Purkinje cell perikarya and molecular layer (left) where the form suggests location in apical dendrites and/or Bergmann glia. ×35

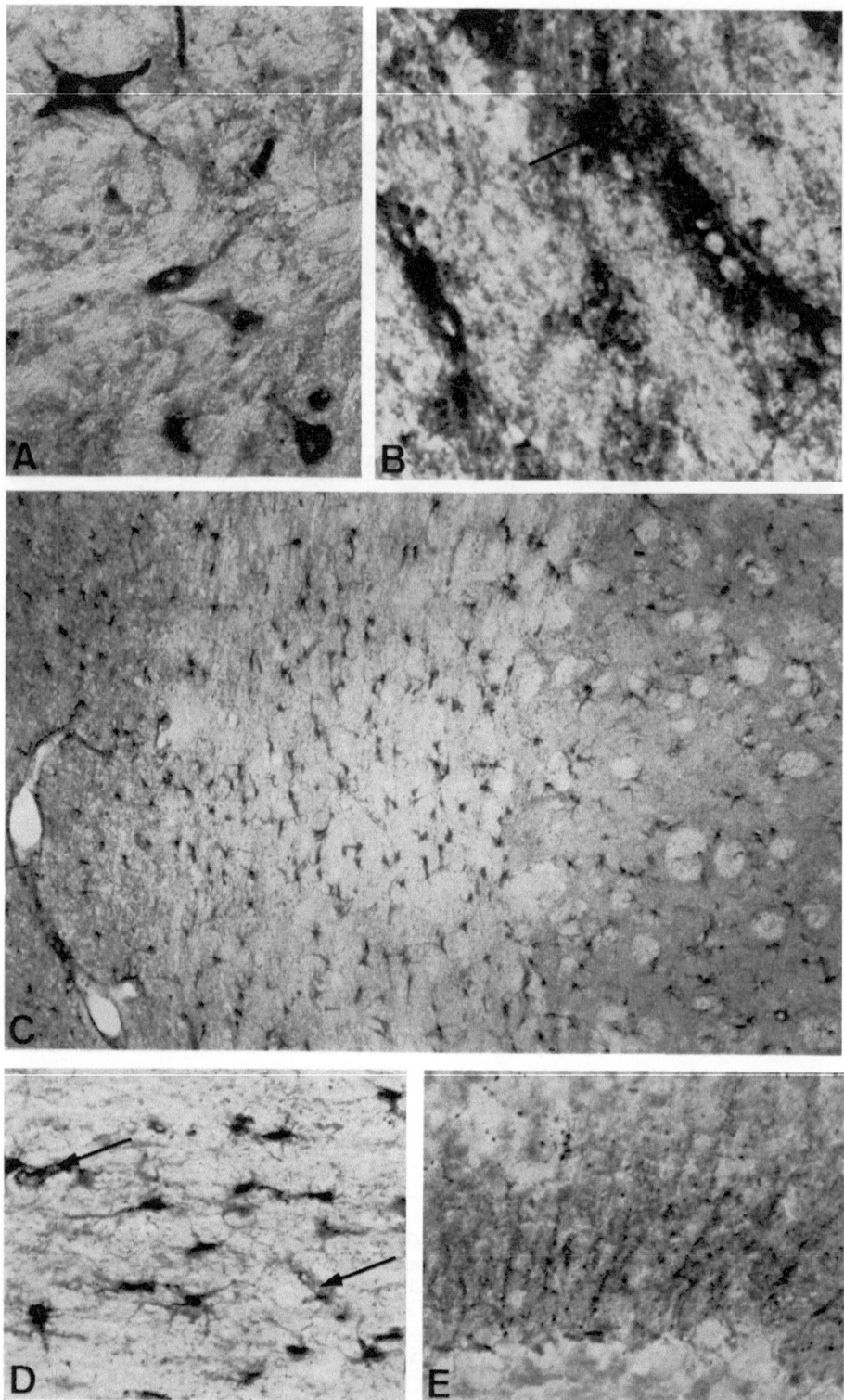

Fig. 3

more greenish and brainstem neurons more prominent (Fig. 3A). Paradoxically, in paraffin sections the neurons were pale while the astrocytes and 'neuropil' were considerably darker (Figs. 3C, D and E); sometimes the same above-mentioned inverse relationship was noted.

These differences in enzymic localization between phosphorylase and phosphorylase + branching enzyme and between either enzyme in cryostat and paraffin sections are not easily explained. However, it was obvious that the medium in *en block* incubation never really reached all elements even on perfusing it; this was probably due to the large molecular size of the components (see Torack, 1965). This difference also explains in part the disparity between the results obtained by different workers (see Table 1). It is obvious, however, that on *en block* incubation phosphorylase + branching enzyme is strongest in neuronal perikarya and processes and in fibrous astrocytes, while phosphorylase alone is localized best in both fibrous and protoplasmic astrocytes. This difference is difficult to reconcile since it is not obvious in cryostat sections.

Although it was mentioned above that glycogen, phosphorylase and branching enzyme generally have the same regional and cytological distribution it is apparent that the method of their demonstration can be responsible for disparity between them, and so can postmortem anoxia, as in the case of white matter (see pp. 8 + 11).

4. Glycogen Synthetase (and Branching Enzyme)

4.1. Biochemical Considerations

The second enzyme capable of the synthesis of α-1,4 linkages of glycogen is glycogen synthetase*. Unlike phosphorylase, it is synthetic both *in vitro* and *in vivo*, it seems to have similar properties in all tissues including CNS, and can not degrade glycogen; it is now proved to be the only synthetic enzyme under normal *in vivo* conditions. It has several features in common with those of phosphorylase,

Fig. 3A—E. Activity of phosphorylase in normal rat brain. A and B are from cryostat cut sections, and stained with dilute Gram's iodine. C, D and E are from paraffin sections and stained with Dimedone-PAS. (A) Large multipolar neurons and "neuropil" of the medullary reticular formation. ×170. (B) Normal white matter (callosal radiation) showing activity in a row of oligodendrocytes (right), an astrocyte (arrow) and "neuropil". The section was overincubated. ×560. (C) Corpus striatum (right), callosal radiation (centre) and frontal cerebral cortex (left). Both protoplasmic and fibrous astrocytes, "neuropil" and vascular walls are positive. ×140. (D) Higher magnification of white matter seen in Fig. 3C with sharply outlined astroglia, vessel walls and astrocytic end feet (arrows), and "neuropil". Note apparent absence of activity in oligodendrocytes and compare with Fig. 3B. ×350. (E) Cerebellar cortex with prominent particulate staining in between relatively pale Purkinje cells. The disposition of the activity suggests location in the Bergmann glia (astrocytes). The molecular layer (above) contains stronger activity than the granular layer (bottom). ×350

* The following summary is based upon articles by Breckenridge and Crawford (1961), Leloir (1964), Larner *et al.* (1968), Manners (1968), Fischer *et al.* (1968), Hers and DeWulf (1968), Goldberg and O'Toole (1969), Goldberg *et al.* (1970), Rottenberg, Passonneau and Lust (1972), Sutherland (1972) and Watanabe and Passonneau (1973).

however. Thus it exists in two forms, an active (I, for independent) and an inactive (D, for dependent); both are interchangeable and regulated by hormonal and nonhormonal factors. The I-form is further activated by G-6-P; at pH 7.0 it doubles the activity and at pH 8.5 it increases it 5-12 fold (Leloir, 1964). Furthermore, the D-form can be transformed to the I-form, not by adding phosphate as in the case of phosphorylase, but by removing it. The enzyme responsible for this is synthetase (transferase)-D-phosphatase. The reverse transformation can also be achieved, and, again, unlike the case of phosphorylase, by a synthetase (transferase)-I-kinase in the presence of ATP. The kinase, as that of phosphorylase, is stimulated by cAMP which, of course, is in turn, influenced by adenyl cyclase and phosphodiesterase and all the factors that influence them. Thus cAMP stimulates *active* phosphorylase formation, but *inactive* glycogen synthetase, formation. "This inverse polarity in a biological sense is a key point..." (Larner et al., 1968). Furthermore, the phosphatase is inhibited nonhormonally by glycogen and the kinase is stimulated by epinephrine through cAMP (Larner et al., 1968), i.e. there is a sort of feed-back control of glycogen synthesis. On the other hand insulin directly stimulates the kinase and hence inhibits glycogen synthesis (Larner et al., 1968). Glucose and glucocorticoids increase by several fold activity of glycogen synthetase, and hence glycogen synthesis, regardless of wheather G-6-P is present or not; this indicated to Hers and De Wulf (1968) that activation of glycogen synthetase by G-6-P is probably of only minor importance in *in vivo* liver. As a matter of fact, in the case of brain glycogen synthetase transformation of D to I forms is apparently not necessary for glycogen synthesis there (Goldberg and O'Toole, 1969). These authors found that giving glucose to diabetic animals, in whose tissues glycogen was double the normal, caused no decrease of UDPG and no increase in glycogen synthetase-I activity; this indicated to them that "glycogenesis in brain can be 'pushed' (e.g. by mass action), whereas it has been shown that in liver it must be 'pulled' (e.g. by synthetase activation to I-form)"! However, anoxia (by decapitation) causes a relative increase (3–4 times) in synthetase-I-form activity (Goldberg and O'Toole, 1969).

The ratio between the activities of 4 enzymes in brain was studied by Breckenridge and Crawford (1961). It turned out that activity of glycogen synthetase is the lowest as compared with that of UDP-glucose pyrophosphorylase, phosphorylase and phosphoglucomutase; $1:12:39:57$, respectively. Nevertheless, the amount of glycogen synthetase present was found sufficient to account for 12 times the normal amount of glycogen.

Glycogen synthetase *in vitro*, like phosphorylase, can not accomplish synthesis of branched glycogen molecules alone but needs a branching enzyme. In this, according to Manners (1968), the process is sequential. a) An existing outer part of a B-chain (main chain) is branched by formation of α-1 → 6-glucosidic linkage to form a new A-chain (side chain); this is accomplished by the branching enzyme which cuts a non-terminal α-1 → 4-glucosidic linkage of a B-chain and reattaches the released chain (usually about 7 residues) by the α-1 → 6-glucosidic linkage, to an A-chain, i.e. the process can be viewed as a transglucosylation in which a chain is transferred from a donor (B-chain) to an acceptor (A-chain). b) The remaining part of the B-chain (stub) is now lengthened by glycogen synthetase activity, i.e. formation of α-1 → 4-linkages, until it can serve as a substrate for branching enzyme again. Hence, glycogen synthetase and branching enzyme act alternately and the glycogen particle contains chains about half of which are

A-chains and contain 6–10 glucose residues, while the rest are B-chains and are usually about 3 times as long (Manners, 1968).

4.2. Histochemical Demonstration

The first method devised for the histochemical visualization of glycogen synthetase activity is that of Takeuchi and Glenner (1961). In their hands it demonstrated good activity in many tissues excepting the CNS; the medium contained UDPG, glycogen, G-6-P, EDTA and tris buffer at pH 7.4. Later however, when he stained the polyglucose product with PAS, Takeuchi (1965 b) was successful in demonstrating a little activity in rat brain. Mossakowski et al. (1967) also demonstrated activity in infant monkey brain; they used the same technique. Sie et al. (1966) modified the medium by increasing the amount of UDPG 4 fold and the G-6-P 45 fold, by adding fluoride and PVP, and by using a higher pH 9.2 (glycine buffer). This medium gave better results in their hands in liver, and in our hands (Ibrahim et al., 1970a, b; Ibrahim et al., 1973) in rat CNS. Sasse (1966) added a step of acid hydrolysis with 10% sulphuric acid to distinguish between preexistant glycogen and newly-synthesized polyglucose. We (Ibrahim et al., 1973), also compared a medium used by Smith (1970) with that of Sie et al., and found it produced inferior results but better than those given by Takeuchi and Glenner's medium; it differed from the latter essentially in containing fluoride which these authors had excluded from their medium because it "impeded the synthesis...".

In all studies, cryostat sections were employed and staining post-incubation was in either Gram's iodine or PAS. We found that localization was poor in brain, although Takeuchi (1965 b) and Mossakowski et al. (1967) did obtain and illustrate better localization. We, therefore, tried en bloc incubation of rat brain as for phosphorylase and, although we ran up against the problem of medium penetration, the intensity of activity and sharpness of localization were greatly improved (Ibrahim et al., 1973).

Electron histochemistry, as mentioned above, has also been used to demonstrate polyglucose synthesis by glycogen synthetase, but in muscle (Takeuchi and Sasaki, 1970).

4.3. Normal Distribution

Although Hutchinson and Kuwabara (1962) expected to find glycogen synthetase in the retina, since they had already found glycogen and phosphorylase, they could not locate any in the normal but the diabetic retina did contain some. Takeuchi (1965 b) reported activity in both grey and white matter of rat brain; white matter and the cerebellar molecular layer were apparently more active. Mossakowski et al. (1967) further found that the enzyme had generally the same distribution as phosphorylase but its activity was weaker; astrocytes were negative, except in the subependymal areas, and the only positive neurons were those of the mesencephalic neucleus of V cranial nerve and the anterior grey horns of the spinal cord. We (Ibrahim et al., 1970a; Ibrahim et al., 1973), confirmed that generally glycogen synthetase has the same distribution as phosphorylase and

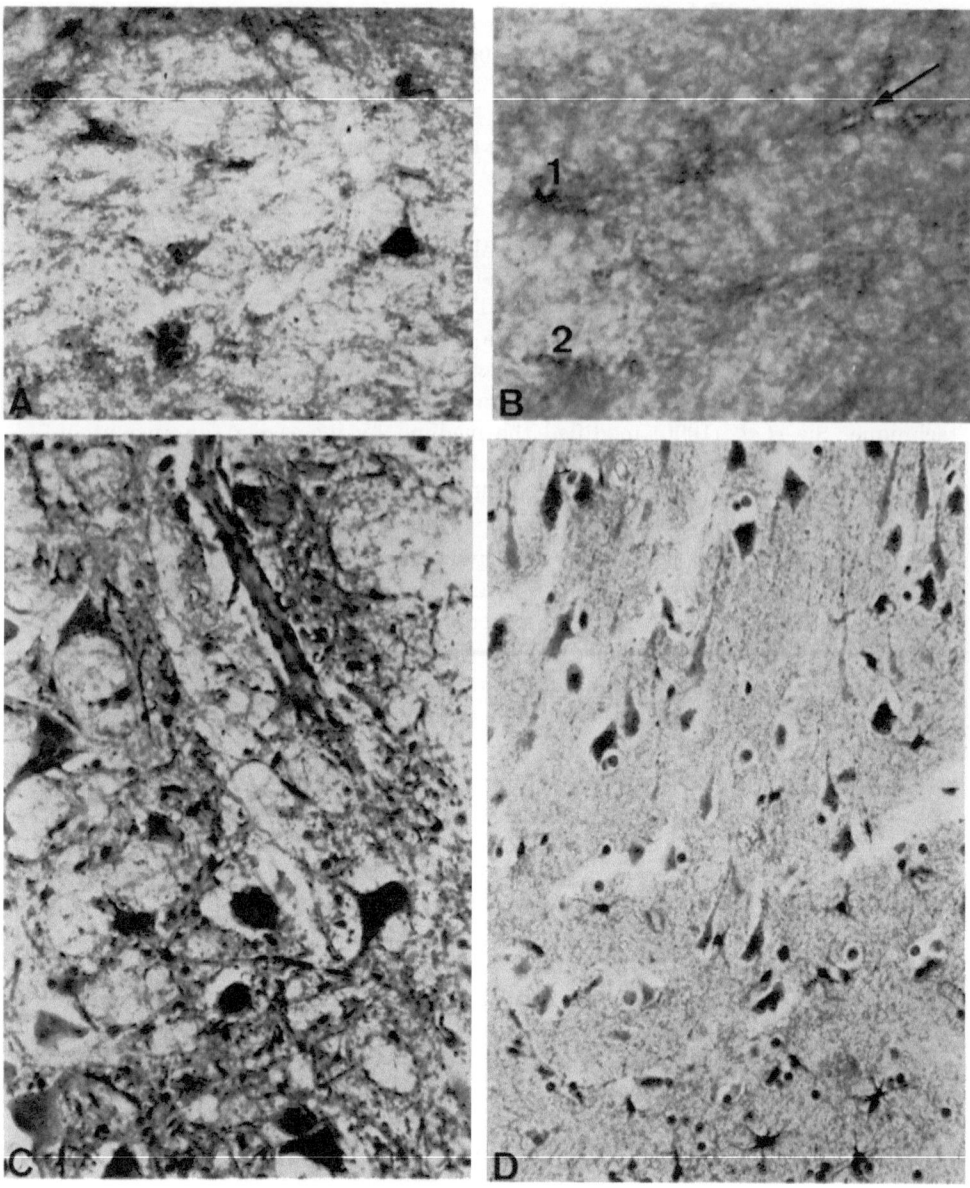

Fig. 4 A—D. Activity of glycogen synthetase in normal rat brain. For the purposes of comparison A and B are from cryostat sections and stained with PAS, while C and D are from paraffin sections, stained with PAS and counterstained with hematoxylin. (A) Reticular formation of medulla with prominent neuronal perikarya and "neuropil". ×140. (B) Hippocampal commissure with poorly-localized activity in an astrocyte (1), a row of oligodendrocytes (2) and a vascular wall (arrow). ×140. (C) Reticular formation of midbrain. Neuronal perikarya, processes, astrocytic end-feet, vascular walls and "neuropil" are positive. ×350. (D) Subiculum of hippocampus (grey matter above) and adjoining alveus (white matter below) show well-localized particulate activity in neurons and diffuse activity in both types of astrocytes, and in "neuropil". Oligodendrocytic enzyme is not apparent. ×350

that the cerebellar molecular layer shows strongest activity; the polyglucose always stained a monochrome brown to purple with iodine indicating its branched nature (see p. 30). PAS gave stronger and sharper localization and, because in this case iodine staining has no advantages over it, was used routinely. Mainly neuronal perikarya and processes, neuropil, astrocytes and smooth muscle of vascular walls showed up (Fig. 4). Although the picture given by paraffin sections was patchy it was usually better than that obtained for phosphorylase and phosphorylase + branching enzyme; all active elements were more sharply delineated. The exception was the oligodendrocytes which, at least in white matter, were visible in cryostat sections but not seen in paraffin sections (Figs. 3 B and 4 D). The reason for this is not clear but it could be that in *en bloc* incubation the oligodendroglial enzyme is either lost or somehow inactivated.

5. Glycogen and its Metabolic Enzymes as a Structural-Functional Unit

A fact critical to the understanding of certain seemingly paradoxical changes in glycogen and its enzymes under pathological conditions is that glycogen and its enzymes, regardless of location, have the same topographic, and often the same cytological distribution, and behave as a structural, as well as a functional, unit. Biochemically, a complex between glycogen and phosphorylase was described by Sutherland and Wosilait in 1956. Since then many other authors have described the same and added to that complex, branching enzyme, glycogen synthetase, synthetase kinase, synthetase phosphatase and phosphorylase phosphatase (Stetten and Stetten, 1960; Selinger and Schramm, 1963; Tata, 1964; Sie et al., 1964; Steiner et al., 1965; Appleman et al., 1966; Rottenberg et al., 1972; Watanabe and Passonneau, 1973). Apparently the bond between glycogen and its related enzymes is much stronger with the granular form and indirect evidence indicates that the active form of phosphorylase is bound preferentially (Tata, 1964). This same intimate relationship has also been demonstrated histochemically both grossly and cytologically in normal heart and liver (Eckner et al., 1968, 1969), normal CNS (Shimizu and Okada, 1957; Ibrahim et al., 1970a), and pathological CNS (Shimizu and Hamuro, 1958; Friede, 1966; Mossakowski et al., 1968; Ibrahim et al., 1968; Nelson et al., 1968; Haymaker et al., 1970; Ibrahim et al., 1970 b; Long et al., 1972).

The importance of this becomes evident when an abnormal glycogen level, say decrease, is accompanied, not by an increase in phosphorylase activity but by a decrease. Normally, one would expect that an increase in phosphorylase activity would be accompanied by a decrease in glycogen, and decrease by an increase, as happens physiologically in normal starved liver (Fagundes and Cohen, 1965; personal observation); upon refeeding, a long-starved liver will, nevertheless, show an increase in the enzymic activity (Niemeyer et al., 1962). The reason for this paradox could be that under abnormal conditions a state might be present where, for example, there is a protracted build-up of glycogen which is also possibly different from the native glycogen and hence has different solubility properties (Leske and Mayersback, 1969) and probably different enzymic susceptibility. Or, it could be that, as is now well-recognized, other factors, beside phosphorylase, can influence glycogenolysis. Thus it is held that nucleotide and inorganic phosphate concentrations are as important as the relative amounts of active and inactive phosphorylases (Parmeggiani and Morgan, 1962; Hornbrook and Brody, 1963; Breckenridge and Norman, 1965; Friede, 1966). Even the changes in various metabolites could influence phosphorylase activity and glycogen metabolism independently and thus help create a paradox. In addition, two tissue enzymes, α-amylase and γ-amylase ("acid" α-glucosidase) are known to effect glycogenolysis (see Rosenfeld, 1964; West et al., 1966). Alpha-amylolysis entails hydrolysis of glycogen to oligosaccharides "which are then broken down to glucose by the action of glucosidases (maltases) one of which, α-1,4-glucosidase (of human liver), hydrolyses not only maltose to glucose but even the external branches of glycogen to glucose" (West et al.). Gamma amylolysis is effected through enzymic splitting of glucose by the breaking of α-1,4-linkages of the glycogen branches, with glucose and γ-dextrins as products (West et al.).

To reestablish equilibrium in a structural-functional unit that has relatively too much glycogen and to initiate more efficient utilization of that glycogen at its new high level in a possibly more glycogen-dependent metabolic state, phosphorylase activity would have to rise; this is the explanation given in simpler form by Prasannan and Subrahmanyam (1968b) in their study of glycogen increase in the alloxan-diabetic rat. Glycogen synthetase activity might increase initially to effect the glycogen accumulation as Long et al. (1972) found in relation to the ischaemic cat spinal cord neurons. We, however, generally found that the increase in glycogen synthetase, if recorded, was increased after both glycogen and phosphorylase. This whole problem is perhaps more complex than this and will be discussed further below.

6. Causes of Glycogen Increase

6.1. Physiological

Normal changes in functional activity can alter the quantity of glycogen present in brain and retina. The normal circadian rhythm effects this so that, for example, brain glycogen (in mouse) is lowest coincident with the peak of locomotor activity and body temperature (Hutchins and Rogers, 1970). This was not found to be the case in the neonate chick in which brain glycogen, although showing a circadian variation, was not apparently closely related to changes in motor activity or body temperature (Edwards and Rogers, 1972).

As mentioned above, the retia changes its glycogen content depending upon the amount of light it is exposed to, i.e. functional activity. Thus the dark-adapted retina contains more glycogen than the one exposed to light and especially in the inner nuclear and outer plexiform layers; this increase over the resting state is assumed to reflect a larger energy reservoir for when the retina is exposed to light and spent ATP, phosphocreatine and acetylcholine need replenishment.

Changes in environmental temperature also influence the glycogen content of brain. In the neonate chick Edwards and Rogers found that a rise in environmental temperature to 40°C caused a depletion of glycogen whereas a decrease to 2°C had no effect. However, a decrease in environmental temperature, severe enough and prolonged enough to affect the body temperature, invariably causes an increase in brain glycogen. Thus in rats a diminution to 18.3°C did that (Svorad, 1958), and in hibernating animals glycogen accumulated in nerve cells, astrocytes, ependyma, choroid plexus (Oksche, 1961), reticular formation, medial thalamic nucleus and tegmentum (Shtark, 1963). Wolff (1968) had confirmed this in the hibernating hedgehog in which considerable aggregates of particulate glycogen accumulated in the large neurons of the supraoptic and paraventricular nuclei and in the "neuropil" of the tuberal nuclei of the hypothalamus; large masses were also seen near the contact areas with the hypophyseal portal capillaries of the infundibular stalk. Recently, Brunner et al. (1971) showed that, in mice, hypothermia caused an increase in brain glycogen. This they attributed to an increase in both blood and brain glucose, presumably secondary to a diminution in metabolic rate. They suggested that the increase in brain was due to (i) increase in activity of the transport mechanism of glucose into brain, and (ii) diminution of cerebral metabolic rate (73% of the normal) and glucose utilization. They also found G-6-P increased and argued that this must have stimulated glycogen synthetase activity (see Leloir, 1968) and inhibited phosphorylase (see Fischer et al., 1968), both of which actions would lead to a glycogen build up; high levels of glucose, per se, inhibit phosphorylase (see Nelson et al., 1968). They concluded nevertheless that the observed levels of G-6-P would not have affected the activity of glycogen synthetase (see Hers and De Wulf, 1968; Goldberg and O'Toole, 1969) although levels of UDPG were lowered indicating that the enzyme's activity was probably increased, but presumably through another mechanism. Nelson et al. (1968) had previously demonstrated similar changes to these when they studied effects of hypothermia as part of a bigger study, and found also that fructose diphosphate was diminished markedly probably reflecting a "decrease in glycolytic flux which (is) in turn a consequence of the decrease in metabolic rate".

Unlike prolonged hypothermia prolonged hyperthermia causes a remarkable depletion of glycogen from all parts of the hypothalamus of the hedgehog (Wolff, 1968).

Hyperglycaemia, per se, in a normal animal (mouse), induced for example by injection of glucose per os, does not cause an increase in brain glycogen but a diminution (Hutchins and Rogers, 1970). In an alloxan-diabetic rat it also does not cause an increase in glycogen of brain (Passonneau et al., 1971). Nevertheless, Shimizu (1954), Friede (1966) and Prasannan and Subrahmanyam (1968 b) have shown that sustained hyperglycaemia does cause an increase in glucose and glycogen of brain; Le Fevre and Peters (1966) and Stewart et al. (1967) found that it increased brain glucose. Still, Edward and Rogers (1972) have found that hyperglycaemia alone, even when sustained for 4 hours in neonate chicks, induced a decrease in brain glycogen rather than an increase. On the other hand, a somewhat longer sustained increase in glucose (6 hr) did cause a 58% increase in glycogen content of adult mouse brain; after only $1^1/_2$ hr exposure no such increase was seen (Nelson et al., 1968). As in the case of hypothermia (Brunner et al., 1971) G-6-P was increased but UDPG was unaffected. Nelson et al. (1968), like Brunner et al., argued that the increase in G-6-P would stimulate glycogen synthesis by stimulating glycogen synthetase but, unlike Brunner et al., they thought that this could also account for the lack of an expected increase in UDPG; Goldberg and O'Toole (1969), who showed that hyperglycaemia does enhance glycogen build-up, found that this was not accompanied by the expected increase in glyco-gen synthetase-I activity (see Hers and De Wulf, 1968). G-6-P would also be expected to inhibit phosphorylase activity (see p. 13). Eventually however, the decreased phosphorylase activity would recover, and even increase, to parallel the increase in glycogen and glycogen synthetase so as to maintain the balance of the glycogen structural-functional unit at a new higher level.

Hypoglycaemia *per se*, generally induced by injection of large doses of insulin, has been reported to affect CNS glycogen in various ways depending on species of animal and age. Thus Edwards and Rogers (1972) found that hypoglycaemia did not alter brain glycogen of neonate chicks, while Hutchins and Rogers (1970) found that in the adult mouse there was a slight diminution (10.7%) after 1 hour, followed by a slight increase (11.2%) after a further hour. On the other hand, Kerr and Ghantus (1936) had found a diminution of glycogen of rabbit brain, and Tews *et al.* (1965) had found that in adult dogs there was a marked drop in cerebral glycogen, as well as in other metabolites such as nucleoside triphosphates, creatine phosphate, lactate, citrate, glutamate and some amino acids. During recovery, up to 1 hour after injecting glucose, most of these metabolites returned to above normal values but glycogen did not. If insulin was given together with glucose (to white mice or rats) a marked rise in cerebral glycogen content occurred and, if the animals had been previously made diabetic by alloxan, insulin + glucose caused an even greater rise in the glycogen (Nelson *et al.*, 1968; Prasannan and Subrahmanyam, 1968a, b; Goldberg and O'Toole, 1969; Passonneau *et al.*, 1971). Of these authors Nelson *et al.* attributed the enhancing effect of insulin to its causing an increase in intracellular glucose and G-6-P concentrations by accelarating glucose transport into the cells. The increase in glucose presumably lead to the increase in G-6-P which caused the increase in glycogen through the mechanisms outlined above; Goldberg and O'Toole, unlike their findings in relation to hyperglycaemia (see above), recorded a 3 fold increase in glycogen synthetase-I activity. Subsequent increase in phosphorylase activity would also occur as mentioned above.

Hypoglycaemia induced by starvation generally caused little or no change in rat brain or retinal glycogen (Kerr and Ghantus, 1936; Kuwabara and Cogan, 1961; Prasannan and Subrahmanyam, 1965); Passonneau *et al.* (1971) reported no change in mice starved overnight. Even when starvation of rabbits was carried until death (Kumamoto, 1953) decrease in brain glycogen was not as much as that of liver; neocortex suffered more loss than archicortex, and areas like the area postrema and subependymal glial tissue hardly suffered at all (see Friede, 1966, p. 142, for more literature review).

6.2. Pathological

Although it is the common practice to find glycogen absent from nearly all routinely processed normal human CNS (see above), glycogen deposits have been, and are being, found with increasing frequency in pathological animal and human CNS. Several authors, some of whom are quoted by Friede (1966), have described many pathological states which are accompanied by glycogen deposits in human CNS, viz. diabetic coma; uraemia; infections or toxic delirium of typhoid; hexachlorophene toxicity (see Lampert *et al.*, 1973); influenza and sepsis; miliary tuberculosis; meningitis and encephalitis; tuberous sclerosis; amaurotic idiocy; poliomyelitis; pernicious anaemia; hepatic encephalopathy; glycogen storage disease; multiple sclerosis; oedematous areas adjacent to certain tumours and infarcts and in areas showing slow frequencies in the EEG (Friede, 1956). In these states most glycogen deposits were in the 'neuropil' in the form of diffuse "dusting" with astrocytic processes often showing the most dense cellular localization. Perivascular spaces, perivascular tissues, subpial tissues and retina also often showed accumulations; reports of neuronal deposits have generally been received with skepticism. Friede does not attempt an explantion of the glycogen increase in these varied and seemingly unrelated conditions.

More recently, Shiraki (1968) has confirmed the increase in glycogen in hepato-cerebral disease, and hepatic failure, in which conditions the abundant glycogen was in the usual sites mentioned earlier, viz. astrocytes, periadventitial spaces of arteries, 'neuropil' and around neurons; he also included intraneural glycogen. Ribadeau-Dumas et al. (1969) have also shown that in cases of Creutzfeldt-Jakob syndrome glycogen deposits in excess of the normal are seen in astrocytes of grey matter; this has quite recently been confirmed by Narang and Field (1973). Furthermore, Watanabe et al. (1973) have reported increases in glycogen content of brain-within astrocytes of a biopsy—of or 3-monthold infant suffering from Pelizaeus-Merzbacher disease. In Pompe's disease (acid α-glucosidase defeciency) there has been described an 8–15 fold increase in glycogen content of cerebral grey and white matter, spinal cord and peripheral nerves (Gambetti et al., 1971; Martin et al., 1973). The glycogen was seen free and membrane-bound in Schwann cells, anterior horn cells, subpial and subependymal zones, astrocytes, maturing oligodendrocytes, ependymal cells, axons, endothelial cells and white blood corpuscles and capillary pericytes. It is of interest that phosphorylase and lysoso-mal acid phosphatase activities were intact while lysosomal α-glucosidase was lacking; the membrane-bound glycogen was suspected to be within lysosomes. This highlights the fact that not all glycogenolysis is due to phosphorylase activity (see p. 34). It is interesting that organelle-located glycogen deposits have also been seen but in mitochondria of reactive types of dystrophic axons (Lampert, 1967). Infantile spongy degeneration has also been shown by Takei and Solitare (1972) to be accompanied by diffuse 'neuropil', as well as perivascular, neuronal and glial glycogen deposits in both grey and white matter. Because glycogen was increased in heart and liver these authors suggested that there was a general disturbance in the biochemical energy supply system. Recently, Fontaine et al. (1973) described glycogen deposits within astrocytes in cases of gangliosidosis similar to Tay-Sachs disease. Finally, it is of interest that Narang and Field (1973) have confirmed older observations of Marinesco (1928) that in multiple sclerosis glycogen deposits are seen in astrocyte processes. Raine et al. (1973) have also noted glycogen accumulation in astrocytes of CNS cultures exposed to diluted serum from multiple sclerosis patients. No suggestion is made as to its etiology.

A pathological state in animals that has been shown to be accompanied by deposits of glycogen is hereditary ataxia of rabbits (Tourtellotte et al., 1966). These workers saw the glycogen in the pons, medulla and midbrain and, although they noted that the amount of glycogen paralleled the severity of the disease, they recorded no significant change in metabolic or glycolytic rates to account for it. They did, however, see an increase in G-6-P in the pons, and cerebellum and an increase in lactate in the pons accompanied by an increase in the cerebellum of glycogen synthetase, phosphorylase and maltase. Nevertheless, because the cerebellum was less affected by disease than the rest of the areas they could not attach much significance to these findings!

6.3. Experimental

Infection with Poliomyelitis Virus

Bodian (1964) has confirmed earlier reports (Marinesco, 1928) of glycogen build-up in human cases of poliomyelitis by showing that glycogen increases in spinal cord of monkeys when these are infected with the Frederich strain of polio virus; this strain has a low neurovirulence. The glycogen was located in chromatolytic neurons and neuroglial processes. This represents a glycogenic response of the neuron to direct injury; in this case by a virus.

Wallerian and Retrograde Degeneration

Indirect injury of the neuron also leads to a glycogen increase. Axotomy (branchial plexotomy) has been shown to cause glycogen accumulation in spinal cord neuronal somata of young chicks (Jirmanová, 1971), while optic nerve sectioning in adult cats was responsible for accumulation of glycogen in presynaptic nerve terminals of optic nerve fibers and in astrocytic processes in the lateral geniculate body (Szentágothai et al., 1966). This reaction was seen as early as 2–4 days after optic nerve section, whereas in the chick neurons maximal glycogen coincided with maximal chromatolytic change, viz. 7th–14th day, but was gone by the 4th week. Jirmanová ascribed the increase in glycogen to its diminished utilization and/or enhanced synthesis, and stressed the young age of the neuron being instrumental in such a reaction. Also, recently Barron et al. (1973) found that retrograde degeneration of rat thalamus induced by unilateral decortiectomy caused the appearance of abnormally large amounts of glycogen in astrocyte processes as well as in neutrophil granulocytes.

Administration of Certain Hormones

It was mentioned above that systemically administered insulin causes hypoglycaemia and either no change or a diminution of brain glycogen, depending on the dosage. However, it should be pointed out here that hypoglycaemia due to insulin is caused secondary to a direct increase in uptake of glucose by the tissues in general. Among these should be the CNS. Nevertheless, because the lowered blood glucose is overwhelmingly more than the expected increase in glucose uptake, the net result is sometimes a diminution in glucose uptake. Since the glycogen stores of CNS are naturally small they start to be used up, and hence, under such circumstances, the glycogen content of CNS decreases. Proof of such a direct effect of insulin on CNS elements was produced by Prasannan and Subrahmanyam (1965) and by Mellerup and Rafaelson (1969) and Mellerup (1970). Prasannan and Subrahmanyam found a 53% increase in brain glycogen of *wellfed* rats when insulin was administered. On the other hand, neither insulin nor glucose alone significantly altered the *fasted* brain glycogen; when glucose was given together with insulin to fasted rats there was a 124% increase in brain glycogen. It is notable that Kerr and Ghantus (1936) found no such increases when glucose, with or without insulin, was administered to rabbits. Mellerup and Mellerup and Rafaelson proved the direct effect of insulin on brain by circumventing its effect on systemic glucose levels by injecting insulin directly intracisternally. However, they tended to believe that the direct effect is not on glucose uptake by the cells, as in muscle and adipose tissue, but is an effect on brain metabolism probably mediated through influence on some enzymic synthesis!

Corticosteroids also influence brain glycogen. Vaccari and Malaguti (1951) found that a large single (narcotic) dose of desoxycorticosterone increased cerebral glycogen 1 hour after injection, whereas an equivalent dose of cortisone caused nothing. Rajan et al. (1963) saw, however, that cortisone, given to fasting rats, did elevate brain glycogen. Timiras et al. (1956) got the same results as Rajan et al. when they used hydrocortisone, and, although glucagon and dextrose, like hydrocortisone, increased blood sugar, these did not increase brain glycogen. These workers attributed the glycogen build-up to the known accelerating effect of hydrocortisone on gluconeogenesis rather than to an inhibiting effect on glucose utilization. On the other hand, Thurston and Pierce (1969) gave repeated doses of hydrocortisone to albino mice and, although they recorded doubling of brain glucose—without increase in blood glucose—they found that both brain glycogen and lactate were unchanged; the increase in brain glucose was attributed to increased permeability or a facilitation of its transport from blood. This observation of a lack of glycogen response was supported later by Mellerup (1970) who showed that intracisternal injection of corticosteroids in rats had no effect on brain glycogen; when the injection was combined with insulin the increase in glycogen was as much as that due to insulin alone. Nevertheless, in the studies by Goldberg and O'Toole (1969) and Watanabe and Passonneau (1973) hydrocortisone did cause an increase in brain glycogen in rats and mice, respectively. Using C^{14}-glucose Watanabe and Passonneau showed, like Thurston and Pierce (1969), increased uptake of glucose by brain from blood and an increase in G-6-P, which might have accounted for increased glycogen synthetase activity and glycogen synthesis. Nevertheless, Goldberg and O'Toole did not record an increase in glycogen synthetase-I activity.

Administration of CNS Depressants

It is now well-established that depression of CNS function by hypnosis (Svorad, 1958), or by drugs, induces an increase in its glycogen content provided their effect is maintained for sufficiently long periods; Kerr and Antaki (1937) found no change in rabbit cerebral glycogen when they administered amytal, evipan, ether and chloroform for only $2^1/_2$–14 min. When some of these anaesthetics were used for 30–60 min there was, however, an increase in cerebral glucose—but not in glycogen—without a concomitant hyperglycaemia; such a response combination, viz. increased cerebral glucose without hyperglycaemia, is regarded as characteristic of the anaesthetic state (Thurston and Pierce, 1969).

The substances studied have included phenobarbitone (Oksche, 1961; Estler, 1961a; Mayman et al., 1964; Gatfield et al., 1966; Nelson et al., 1968; Hutchins and Rogers, 1970; Folbergrová et al., 1970; Ibrahim et al., 1970a; King et al., 1973; Hoffmann et al., 1973; Watanabe and Passonneau, 1973; Macmillan and

Siesjö, 1973), ether (Estler and Heim, 1960; Mayman *et al.*, 1964; Pronaszko-Kurczyńska *et al.*, 1971; Passonneau *et al.*, 1971; Brunner *et al.*, 1971), ethanol (Eletskii, 1963; Ammon *et al.*, 1965; Roach and Reese, 1971; Veloso *et al.*, 1972), chlorpromazine (Estler, 1961b; Mayman *et al.*, 1964; Hutchins and Rogers, 1970; Koizumi and Shiraishi, 1970), reserpine (Albrecht, 1957; Hutchins and Rogers, 1970), meprobamate (Estler, 1961b; Hutchins and Rogers, 1970), chloroform (Mayman *et al.*, 1964), halothane (Brunner *et al.*, 1971; Husain and Paradise, 1973), methoxyflurane and ethrane (Brunner *et al.*, 1971), haloperidol and phenylbutazone (Hutchins and Rogers, 1970), and thalidomide (Estler, 1961b).

Research into the biochemical mechanisms underlying glycogen increase due to phenobarbitone has been the most extensive. Estler (1961a), for instance, recorded a fall in body temperature during phenobarbital anaesthesia but concluded that the increase in glycogen was not due to the lowering of the body temperature but to the sedative effect. The glucose content of brain was doubled during anaesthesia with phenobarbitone, as well as with chloroform and ether; chlorpromazine caused only small increases in the glucose (Mayman *et al.*, 1964). Like some authors, Mayman *et al.* found an increase in blood glucose and attributed the raised glucose and new glycogen of brain partly to this and partly to a slowing metabolic rate of brain. The conclusions of Nelson *et al.* (1968) would agree with this and add the possible role of the increased G-6-P (see p. 36). Nelson *et al.* further suggested that the decrease in inorganic phosphate, which they had reported earlier, would similarly lower phosphorylase activity.

Therefore, a decreased metabolic rate in the presence of an increased glucose, activated glycogen synthetase and decreased phosphorylase activity would all together account for the glycogen buildup. Folbergrová *et al.* (1970) have confirmed that phenobarbital anaesthesia decreases metabolic rate in brain, both grey and white matter and more so the latter, which, as mentioned above, they found to normally have 30% higher glucose and a higher metabolic rate than grey matter. All the rest of the above-mentioned authors agree that the metabolic rate of brain is decreased by CNS depressants (see Hultborn and Jarlstedt, 1974). Strangely, Pontén *et al.* (1973), working with nitrous oxide anaesthesia, concluded that, "neither superficial nor deep anaesthesia affect the energy state of the rat cerebral cortex, as evaluated from the tissue concentrations of ATP, ADP or AMP ..."

The studies by Ibrahim *et al.* (1970a), Watanabe and Passonneau (1973) and Husain and Paradise (1973) need special mention here because they included direct evidence of neosynthesis of glycogen. Ibrahim *et al.* demonstrated histologically an increase in glycogen granules in sites of rat brain normally showing glycogen, whereas Watanabe and Passonneau and Husain and Paradise showed an increase in glycogen in mouse brain by studying uptake of C^{14} glucose. Watanabe and Passonneau also found that the ratio of phosphorylase a to total phosphorylase was markedly decreased while the ratio of glycogen synthetase I to total synthetase was not affected. They thus concluded that the 2.5 fold increase in glycogen they observed was due to a decrease in the rate of phosphorolysis rather than to an elevation in glycogenesis. The persistence of glycogen in spite of the subsequent increase in phosphorylase, which was previously observed by Passonneau and co-workers (Nelson *et al.*, 1968), was attributed to the possibility that not all glycogen of brain is available to the phosphorylase; they had shown that glycogen of brain is bound to glycogen synthetase and suggested that such bound glycogen is not fully available to the phosphorylase. According to Husain and Paradise halothane blocked an early step in glycolysis preceding phosphofructokinase, glucose uptake or glucose phosphate isomerization to fructose phosphate; higher doses than those clinically employed inhibited the electron transport process.

Narcosis of ether differs from that induced by phenobarbitone in that ether has a sympathomimetic action, with liver glycogenolysis and hyperglycaemia obviously manifest (Brunner et al., 1971; Passonneau et al., 1971). Although other anaesthetics mentioned above, including ethanol, have no such sympathomimetic effect yet all cause hyperglycaemia and an increase in brain glucose even higher than that of blood (Mayman et al., 1964; Brunner et al., 1971; Passonneau et al., 1971), this presumably being due to (1) either a stimulating effect on the carrier-mediated glucose transport system (Mayman et al., 1964), or an increased permeability to glucose, plus (2) a diminution of cerebral metabolic rate and glucose utilization. The increased glucose and diminished metabolic rate would cause the increase in glycogen through the same mechanisms outlined above.

The mode of action of the sedative drugs is in all probability, generally the same as described for the anaesthetics. Thus for instance, chlorpromazine was found to cause a small increase in blood and brain glucose (Mayman et al., 1964) as well as an inhibition of glycolytic metabolism (Koizumi and Shiraishi, 1970).

Diminution of Brain Biogenic Amines

This could be achieved by the injection of drugs that cause depletion of these amines, e.g., serpasil (Albrecht, 1957), drugs that are blockers of β-adrenergic receptors, e.g. propranolol (Estler and Ammon, 1966, 1967; Somerville and Smith, 1972) or many CNS depressants mentioned above (Hutchins and Rogers, 1970), and possibly the CNS stimulants caffeine and cocaine (Hutchins and Rogers, 1970). Convulsions caused by methionine sulphoximine injection (Folbergrová et al., 1969; Folbergrová, 1973), or electroshock (Shimizu and Kubo, 1957; see also Freide, 1966, p. 142) also cause a glycogen build-up. Sympathectomy, chemically induced by injecting 6-hydroxydopamine (Passonneau et al., 1971), or deprivation of a part of the brain (caudate nucleus) of its afferent monoamine supply (dopamine mainly but also a little 5-HT and noradrenaline, Hoffmann et al., 1973) again induces an increase in glycogen in the deafferented parts. This is evidence in support of the belief that the glycogen content of a tissue may be in part regulated by its autonomic nerve supply (Hoffmann et al., 1973); this had, in fact, been observed previously in relation to liver of rabbit (Shimizu, 1967) and cardiac muscle of cat (Daw and Berne, 1967). In all of these instances it is the adenyl cyclase system that is affected by the monoamine deprivation (see Mršulja, 1974). This, in turn, causes a diminution in cAMP content. Since, as mentioned above, cAMP normally stimulates synthesis of active phosphorylase and inactive glycogen synthetase D, the net result of its decrease would be, as expected, an increase in glycogenesis and a decrease in glycogenolysis with resultant glycogen build-up.

Understandably therefore, sympathectomy by 6-hydroxydopamine was found to cause a decrease in glucose and an increase in glycogen of mouse brain; UDPG was unexpectedly increased however (Passonneau et al., 1971). Shimizu (1967) had shown the same sort of changes on parasympathetic stimulation of rabbit liver, but Daw and Berne (1967) had failed to detect the expected increase in active glycogen synthetase I and inactive phosphorylase b in chronically sympathectomized cat heart; phosphorylase was not significantly altered. Folbergrová (1973), studying the effects of methionine sulphoximine, also found no change in total phosphorylase but phosphorylase a was reduced by 50%. This meant a decrease in glycogenolysis, but they believed that an increase in glycogenesis was most likely as well. The glycogenic effect of propranolol was also attributed to a decrease in phosphorylase activity; there is no mention of glycogen synthetase (Estler and Ammon, 1966, 1967). However, these authors added as well two other probable factors, viz., a direct inhibitory effect on the glycolytic enzyme system and a reduction of energy requirements and carbohydrate metabolism by blockade of the β-receptors. It should be added here that the recent study of Schultz and Daly (1973) involves the α-receptors more than the β-receptors in the enhancement of cAMP synthesis.

Irradiation

Klatzo et al. (1961) were the first to demonstrate that glycogen accumulates in rat brain following irradiation with ionizing (alpha) particles. With high doses (6000 rad), and animals killed from 5 min to 5 months after irradiation, they found that glycogen granules appeared in the irradiated parts of the brain and were located in glial cells some 12 hr postradiation. Obvious breakdown of the bloodbrain barrier (BBB), shown by leakage of fluorescent-labelled material, was noted later, some 48 hr postradiation. This long delay in the breakdown of the BBB does not, of course, reflect the real speed with which membrane permeability breaks down since Rothenberg (1950) and others have shown that after irradiation breakdown occurs at the ionic level (Na^+, K^+, Ca^{++}) in a matter of minutes (see also Ginsburg and Ulmer, 1958; Loutit, 1952; Bresciani et al., 1964; Köver and Schoffeniels, 1966). On the basis of their findings, Klatzo et al. concluded that disturbance in vascular permeability plays a secondary role to direct physical injury of cellular mechanisms by alpha-particles (see Haymaker, 1970). They suggested that the glycogen increase might be due to release of protein-bound glycogen from damaged tissues followed by its uptake and accumulation in the glial cells.

A little later, this group of workers (Miquel et al., 1963) found similar aggregates of glycogen in brains of X-irradiated rats. They concluded then that the mechanism of glycogen increase "may consist in an impairment of the enzymes mediating the incorporation and release of glucose from glycogen". Later still, Miquel and Haymaker (1965) analysed four possible mechanisms for glycogen accumulation: "1. liberation of carbohydrate in the injured tissue and its subsequent uptake by glial cells, 2. increase in permeability of the BBB to glucose, 3. inhibition of the process of anaerobic glycolysis, and 4. inhibition of aerobic glycolysis." Initially, they favoured the second possibility but their final conclusion, supported later by Kay and Chan (1967), was in favour of the fourth; it should be remembered, however, that inhibited aerobic glycolysis per se only stimulates anaerobic glycolysis and can not lead to glycogen build-up. This apparently mainly applied to "the astroglia-neuron metabolic unit" because glycogen had accumulated in astroglia. Stress was laid on the transport by astroglia of fluid, ions, and glucose. Derangement of such functions by irradiation could possibly lead to accumulation of glycogen in the astroglia. Predominance of glycogen in the protoplasmic astrocytes, in contrast to its scarcity in the fibrous astrocytes of white matter, was considered a reflection of differences in their metabolic behaviour (Miquel and Haymaker, 1966). However, evidence was seen of alteration of neuronal metabolism under these conditions which might have suggested influence on the closely associated protoplasmic, but not the independent, fibrous astroglia.

Histochemical studies of enzyme activities related to glycogen metabolism in irradiated animals were first undertaken and later expanded by us (Ibrahim et al., 1968; Ibrahim et al., 1970a). In young adult rats exposed to whole body X- or gamma-rays, phosphorylase activity of the brain was noted to increase as early as 3 hr postradiation to a maximum at 8–18 hr. A gradual decrease began after the second day but abnormally high activity was still present on the sixth day. In general, the increase in phosphorylase activity paralleled that in glycogen, although, for unknown reasons, the enzymic activity returned to normal more slowly than did the glycogen content.

Increases in both glycogen and phosphorylase occurred in all locations normally containing glycogen (see above and Figs. 5A and B), and also in areas normally apparently devoid of it, such as some layers of the olfactory bulb, deeper five layers of the neocortex, thalamic nuclei, some molecular layers of the hippocampus, central white matter (corpus callosum and callosal radiations) and olfactory tracts, but only with the highest dose given (10500 R gamma-rays) and maximally in regions closely adjacent to grey matter (see Fig. 5A and Ibrahim et al., 1970a). As in previous studies, the neurons showed no obvious changes in glycogen or phosphorylase. Both increased glycogen granules and phosphorylase activity were generally in the same elements, viz. astrocytes, the "neuropil" and, with higher doses, the griseal oligodendrocytes (see Ibrahim et al., 1970a). One salient exception to this was the oligodendrocytes of the white matter which often showed increased enzyme activity but not increased glycogen; only the highest dose caused the appearance of sparse glycogen granules in these cells. This apparent discrepancy could be accounted for by the greater and faster utilization of glycogen by white matter that was mentioned earlier. Glycogen synthetase was largely unchanged and, of several oxidoreductive enzymes tested, only activity of hexokinase and 6-phosphogluconate dehydrogenase was apparently increased in astrocytes at $1/2$–2 hr and 24 hr respectively.

The principal findings from our studies include the following: 1. An increase in glycogen in areas normally showing it but especially in some "vulnerable" sites (see Hypoxia and Ischaemia; Miquel and Haymaker, 1965; Ibrahim et al., 1968, 1970a). 2. The often simultaneous increase in phosphorylase, both active and total, in the same sites as those of glycogen increase. 3. The almost parallel temporal changes in glycogen content and phosphorylase. 4. The apparently unchanged activity of glycogen synthetase and some oxidoreductive enzymes, with moderate increases in hexokinase and 6-phosphogluconate dehydrogenase.

The significance of the vulnerability of certain sites to glycogen accumulation lies in their similarity to vulnerable sites in the other experimental conditions to be discussed. Simultaneous increases in glycogen and phosphorylase in the same areas, and even in the same cell, emphasize the intimate relationship mentioned above between glycogen and its enzymes.

The mechanisms through which glycogen increase occurred could be:

1. Hyperglycaemia, a common feature of whole body but not of head alone irradiation (Kay and Entenman, 1956; Kay and Chan, 1967; Lundgren and Miquel, 1970), leads to abnormally high levels of glucose in brain. This rise in

glucose is probably enhanced by the greater glucose permeability of X-irradiated cells (Wesemann *et al.*, 1962). Increased glucose in metabolically intact brain can *per se* cause glycogen accumulation (see p. 35).

2. Both aerobic and anaerobic glycolysis in brain are diminished owing to several factors. There is decreased activity of glyceraldehyde-3-phosphate dehydrogenase (G-3-PD) and adenosine triphosphatase both of which enzymes are-SH ones (Filipova and Seits 1964; Köver and Schoffeniels, 1966). Also, synthesis of coenzyme A (Trufanov and Popova, 1956) and active acetate (Filipova and Seits, 1964) is diminished. Again, soon after irradiation the concentration of nicotinamide adenine dinucleotide (NAD), on which anaerobic glycolysis depends, falls (Maas and Schubert, 1958). On the basis of these changes, inhibition of both forms of glycolysis would be expected and does occur (Egaña, 1962); aerobic metabolism has also been reported to be directly damaged (Frank and Snezhko, 1961; Kay and Chan, 1967).

3. Membrane permeability of cells and their organelles is altered (Franke and Lierse, 1966). This, plus direct damage to the sodium pump (Loutit, 1952; Bresciani *et al.*, 1964; Köver and Schoffeniels, 1966), presumably caused by inhibition of the Na^+-K^+-stimulated ATPase (Köver and Schoffeniels, 1966; Filipova and Seits, 1964), would cause diminution of ATP utilization, and hence ATP build-up, with consequent reversal of the normal glycolytic pathway. It would also cause accumulation of Na^+ (Rothenberg, 1950) and loss of K^+ (Ginsburg and Ulmer, 1958). The latter effect could add to the inhibition of glycolysis since K^+ stimulates brain (Ashford and Dixon, 1935) and mitochondrial respiration (Papa *et al.*, 1965) probably through its action on the Embden-Meyerhof pathway (DePiras and Zadunaisky, 1965), as well as the citric acid cycle (Tsukada and Takaguchi, 1955). Membrane permeability and ionic changes are probably the direct causes of oedema which appears in X-irradiated rabbit brain, mild up to 8–12 hr but more severe thereafter (Gerstner *et al.*, 1956; Gerstner and Kent, 1957).

4. A rise in brain 5-HT, as has been described following X-irradiation (Nair, 1965), and release of 5-HT from its widespread binding sites in the brain (Renson and Fischer, 1959; Melching, 1965; Nair, 1965; Palaić and Supek, 1966) may contribute to the membrane damage and hence to the oedema above-mentioned; release of other monoamines is also possible. A similar rise of 5-HT in irradiated intestine has been implicated in the causation of oedema there (Willoughby, 1960; Detrick, 1963). Such oedema would further impair transport mechanisms across all membranes, and also tissue oxygenation (Levine and Klein, 1960), with impediment of aerobic and, eventually anaerobic, glycolysis. However, release from its binding sites, and perhaps increase, of 5-HT in brain would probably stimulate the activity of the adenyl cyclase system leading to activation of phosphorylase with consequent increased glycogenolysis (see p. 14); this would naturally, at least partially, counterbalance the effect on vascular permeability and glycolysis. On the other hand, release of 5-HT, as its injection experimentally, would cause widespread vasoconstriction, haemostasis, platelet destruction and further release of 5-HT, thus introducing an element of ischaemia with its consequences (see p. 69; Ibrahim, 1972; Welch *et al.*, 1973; Allen *et al.*, 1974; Wurtzman and Zervas, 1974).

All of the above factors converge on inhibition of glycolysis as the direct cause of glycogen accumulation, a conclusion in accord with the view of most warkers cited above. Abnormally high glucose concentrations in a brain incapable of metabolizing it must enhance the build-up further. The increase observed in 6-phosphogluconate dehydrogenase activity may indicate hyperactivity of the direct oxidative pathway as a compensatory reaction to impeded glycolysis via the Embden-Meyerhof pathway. An apparent lack of change in other oxidoreductive enzyme activities must be regarded with caution however, for histochemical results, unless quantitated, can be misleading.

It is of interest that recently Calvo and Forteza-Vila (1972) found that whole body X-irradiation of rats induces an increase in glycogen of peripheral nerves in bone marrow. This was seen in myelinated and unmyelinated axons (30% of all axons) and Schwann cells, 1–30 days postradiation. It is curious that in normal animals these authors found 6% of non-myelinated axons showed glycogen whereas myelinated fibers showed none.

Direct Trauma

Several reports have described glycogen accumulation in areas of CNS directly traumatized by mechanical means (stab wound) (Friede, 1953, 1962, 1966; Hess, 1955; Shimizu and Hamuro, 1958; Oksche, 1961; Smith et al., 1966; Hager et al., 1967; Ibrahim et al., 1968; Guth and Watson, 1968; Klatzo et al., 1970; Haymaker et al., 1970; Noak et al., 1971; Farkas-Bargeton et al., 1972; Bignami and Dahl, 1974); a report on a similar effect due to injury by a laser beam has also appeared (Lampert et al., 1966), and so have two reports on the effects of trauma caused by the locol application of cold to the branis of rats (Blakemore, 1969) and cats (Long et al., 1973) in which reactive astrocytes showed increased glycogen.

Generally, in these studies the trauma was inflicted on young adult rat brains which were examined at various intervals thereafter; Farkas-Bargeton et al. (1972) also used infant rats. All workers described zonation in the stab area: A central (innermost) coagulum zone containing clotted blood is surrounded by an intermediate necrotic tissue zone and then follows an outermost transition zone which blends imperceptibly with normal brain matter. It is the transition zone that contains the glycogen deposits present mainly perivascularly, in "neuropil" and in somewhat swollen (oedematous) astrocytes, especially those of grey matter. Biochemically, the increased glycogen is not confined to the site of injury; using a quantitative micromethod Guth and Watson (1968) have found that the increased glycogen was throughout the injured cerebral hemisphere and that small amounts were present even in the contralateral hemisphere.

The glycogen was generally first observed in the adult rats about 6 hr after the trauma, but Klatzo et al. (1970) were able to find noticeable amounts only $2^1/_2$ hr after trauma. However, Klatzo et al. (1970) and Farkas-Bargeton et al. (1972) did not record any increase in glycogen in 4–13 day-old rats; 28–150 day-old ones did show considerable glycogen. The excess glycogen was observed until 4–5 days, thereafter gradually disappearing over 2 weeks (Guth and Watson, 1968). Hager et al. (1967) could, however, still detect excess glycogen in the astroglia by electron microscopy until 4 months after injury. It is of interest that biochemically they found the increase restricted to the bound form of glycogen whereas free glycogen content remained normal. Glycogen content of neurons in the severely-damaged zones was lost while in the zone of glycogen excess it was unchanged or slightly increased, especially in cerebral cortical neurones of 21 day old rats one day after trauma (Ibrahim, unpublished observations).

The lack of glycogen increase in the 4–13 day-old rats is of interest because the normal brains of this age group actually contain more glycogen, and have a lower oxygen consumption, as compared with the older rats (Farkas-Bargeton et al., 1972). These authors attributed the lack of glycogen increase to the "paucity and non-reactivity of astrocytes...". It is of further interest that newly-hatched chicks, like infant rats and mice, also do not respond to sustained hyperglycaemia by a glycogen build-up (Edwards and Rogers, 1972; see p. 35).

Inquiry into the mechanism(s) underlying glycogen increase lead Guth and Watson (1968) to suggest three possibilities: 1. Injured tissue liberates carbohydrate, which is then taken up by glial cells and stored as glycogen. 2. Increased systemic supply of glucose, with increased permeability to it, raises intracellular glucose. 3. Decreased aerobic and/or anaerobic glycolysis does the same as in (2). Later, Guth, working with Klatzo et al. (1970), used H^3- and C^{14}-glucose incorporation and concluded that the glycogen increase was triggered by "oversupply of glucose which otherwise is not being utilized at the normal rate"; the glycogen increase would then be due to a "step-up in synthesis" rather than to a decrease in breakdown. This conclusion, they thought, was supported by the fact that in their previous studies on asphyxia of neonate monkeys (Mossakowski et al., 1968) they had noted an increase in glycogen synthetase activity in astrocytes of actively meylinating white matter. The logic of this escapes us since their conclusion obviously implicates a decrease in utilization of glucose which, unable to escape, would have to be stored in the form of glycogen; an increase in glycogen synthetase activity may then become necessary. Klatzo et al. do in fact ultimately reach a similar conclusion not only in relation to trauma but also to radiation, anoxia and ischaemia in which, as mentioned earlier, they envisage neurons primarily and the related astrocytes, which transmit nutritive glucose, secondarily involved (see Miquel and Haymaker, 1965). They found, however, that such a concept fails to explain glycogen accumulation in white matter astrocytes, in oligodendrocytes and in some neurons under certain conditions such as hibernation (see p. 35) and ischaemia (see p. 55).

As might be expected, oxidoreductive enzyme activity (cytochrome oxidase, succinate dehydrogenase and NADH-dehydrogenase) was lost, or greatly reduced, in the necrotic zone and its immediate vicinity (Shimizu and Hamuro, 1958; Friede, 1962; Farkas-Bargeton et al., 1972; Robinson, 1973). Shimizu and Hamuro (1958), Ibrahim et al. (1968) and Farkas-Bargeton et al. (1972) also described a similar decrease in phosphorylase in the same areas; however, an increase in phosphorylase and alkaline phosphatase accompanied the increase in glycogen in young adult rat brain. Shimizu and Hamuro, Friede, and Ibrahim et al., all suggested that the increase in glycogen was due to lowered metabolic rates.

To elucidate sequential, enzymic, distributional and aetiological factors operative in the glycogen accumulation caused by direct trauma we inflicted several types of unilateral injury on brains of rats, viz. deep incision either coronally or sagitally placed, isolation of an olfactory bulb from its hemisphere or destruction of the cerebellar cortex. In some instances even the seemingly slight trauma of thinning the bone with a drill over areas of the cerebral cortex induced glycogen accumulation. The animals were killed at varying intervals.

Although several structures were usually damaged, not all of them showed increase in glycogen. For example, following incisions about the level of the optic chiasm (Fig. 6), the neocortex, molecular layers of the hippocampus and the thalamus contained much glycogen, adjacent areas less and others not at all. As found in the other two experimental models discussed *in extenso* in this review certain areas were "vulnerable" or "sensitive" and could show glycogen accumulation, while others were less sensitive and hence refractory to glycogen accumulation (compare Figs. 5A, 6B, C and 10A). However, "low sensitivity" areas directly adjacent to incision did contain glycogen deposits analogous to high doses of ionizing radiation (see p. 43). The distribution of glycogen in the cerebral cortex was very extensive (Fig. 6A–C) and almost co-extensive with it was the distribution of the markers of oedema-Evans blue and sodium fluorescein—when these were used (Fig. 6B, C and E).

In all instances, there were the various zones mentioned above (Fig. 6A, B and D). Within the coagulum zones there were usually masses of polymorphonuclear neutrophil leukocytes heavily laden with glycogen (Fig. 6A); at some distance in the brain substance, extravasated neutrophils were also glycogen laden but intravascular ones were not. The extent of the glycogen-bearing zones depended on the site and degree of damage inflicted (Fig. 6A and B). Thus a small cerebellar lesion induced glycogen deposition only in the cortces of neighbouring folia, and the glycogen-bearing zone formed an arc of a circle (a "front") with the necrotic zone at its geometric centre. Cerebellar nuclei, unless reached by the "front", were free of glycogen, as were intervening areas of white matter, which were however oedematous (see Haymaker *et al.*, 1973, Fig. 3). Similar lesions were seen in limited destruction of the olfactory bulb (Fig. 6A).

Extensive destruction induced glycogen at great distances from the insult site. For instance, in lesions at the olfactory bulb almost the entire ipsilateral neocortex and often the amygdaloid nuclei and the pyriform and entorrhinal corteces showed excess glycogen (Fig. 6A and C). Oligodendroglial and microglial hypertrophy (Fig. 7A and B) and swollen and glycogen-laden astrocytes were seen at these sites (Fig. 7C). Review of the anatomical connections of the rhinencephalon indicated that these changes could have partly arisen as a reaction to stimuli generated at the site of injury. Furthermore, the degree of backward and lateral extension of the reaction seemed to parallel the extent of the necrosis. To test the possible influence of Wallerian, retrograde or transneuronal degeneration on glycogen content, the lateral geniculate bodies of cats were examined 24 hr after unilateral destruction of their occipital cortices. In addition, lateral geniculate ganglia and visual cortices of rats were examined up to 3 months after unilateral eye enucleation. Both experiments, were however unsuccessful in eliciting glycogen excesses, the former probably owing to its short duration and the latter to the insensitivity of the lateral geniculate body to glycogen accumulation, as supported by the irradiation and hypoxia experiments. Somewhat comparable experiments performed by Glees *et al.* (1967) and by Barron and Doolin (1968) were equally unsuccessful, probably for the same reasons. However, a similarly designed experiment on the cat cerebellum did show glycogen deposits in astrocytes of cerebellar roof nuclei upon damage of the overlying cortex; this took $3^{1}/_{2}$ months to appear (Eager and Eager, 1966). Also, a similar experiment involving occipital cortiectomy in the monkey demonstrated delayed increase in size and number of astrocytes, microglia and oligodendrocytes accompanying eventual loss of neurons from the ipsilateral lateral geniculate body; the status of glycogen was not mentioned (Mihailović *et al.*, 1971).

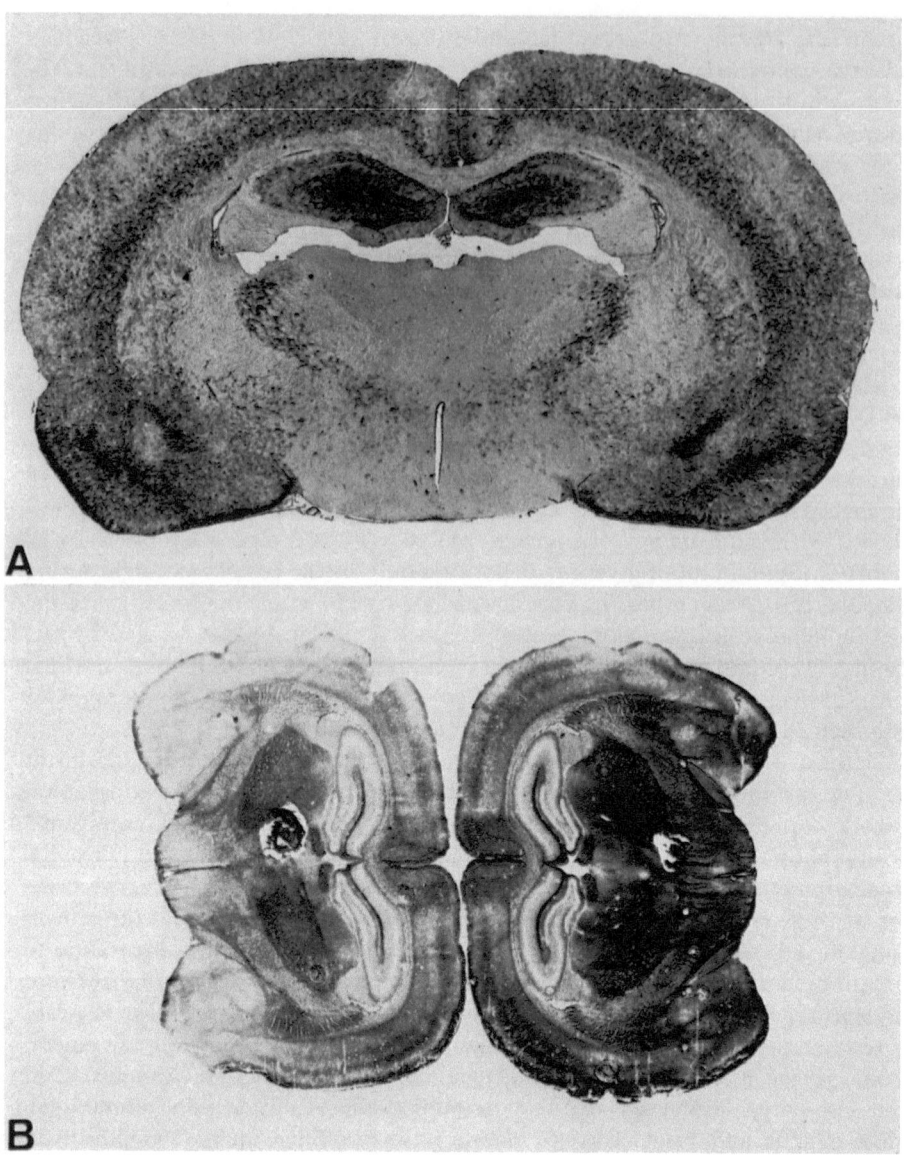

Fig. 5. (A) Brain of a rat exposed 24 hr previously to 10500 r γ-rays. Glycogen deposits are heavy in and around areas normally rich in it being maximal in dentate gyrus of hippocampal formation, amygdaloid complex, pyriform cortex and lateral thalamus; the corpus callosum and callosal radiations show some glycogen. The normal brain at this magnification shows no glycogen. Dimedone-PAS, ×8. (B) Brain of a rat exposed to 2000 r X-rays 48 hr before sacrifice (right) beside a normal (control) brain. Note generalized increase in total phosphorylase activity which is generally especially marked in areas corresponding to those with most glycogen in (A). Increase in white matter activity is just discernible. Dilute Gram's iodine, ×4.2

Fig. 6. (A) Brain of a rat in which the left hemisphere was incompletely transected just posterior to the olfactory bulb 24 hr prior to sacrifice. The right half of the brain is used as control but small amounts of glycogen deposits are seen there also, especially in the outer cerebral cortex. The most anterior dark mass consists of blood elements (mostly PAS-positive neutrophil leukocytes). Note that the circular shape of the glycogen "front" is interrupted in the region of the corpus rallosum (arrow). Dimedone-PAS-gallocyanin, ×3.4. (B) Same as in

48

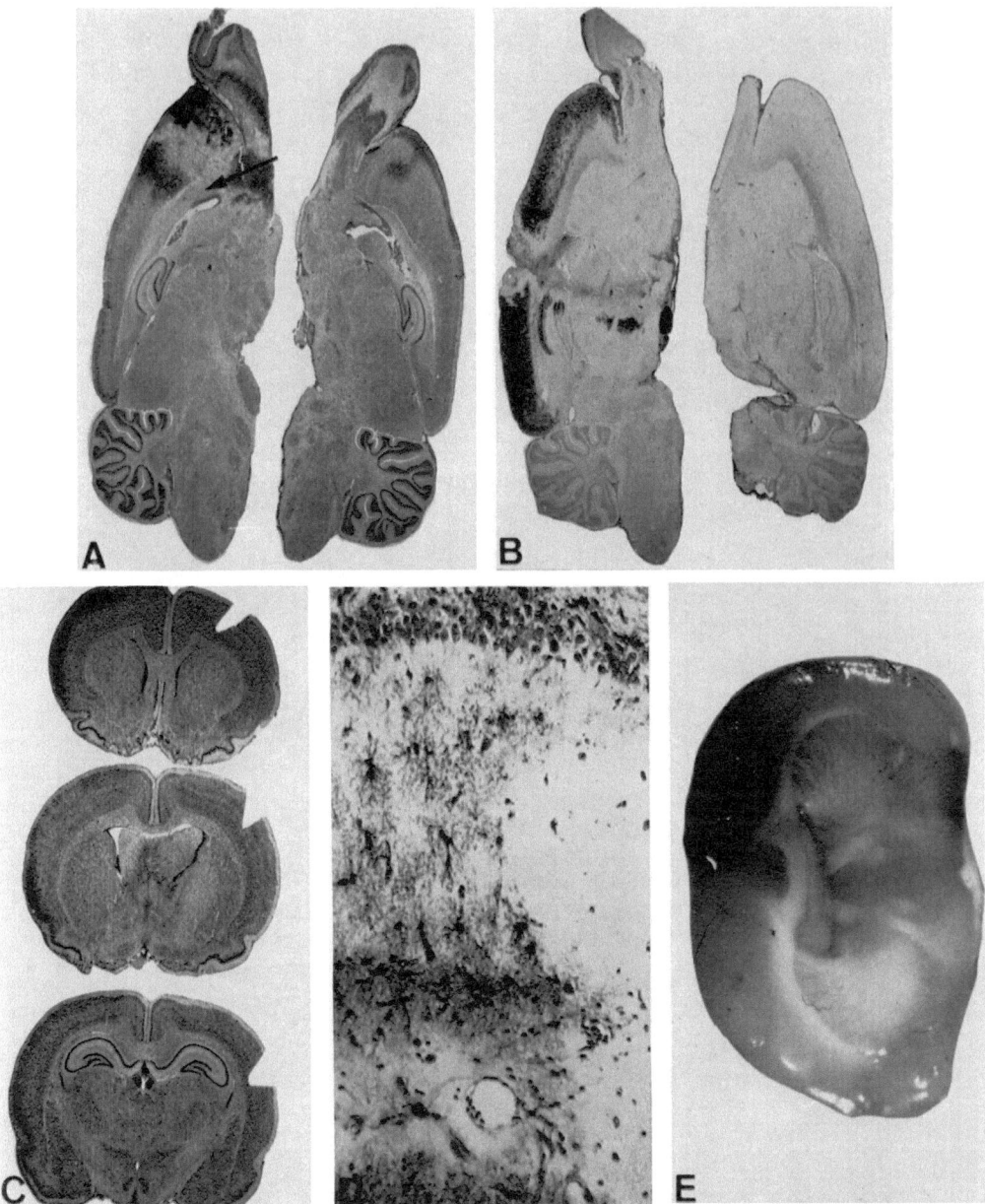

Fig. 6 A except that the wound was inflicted further back. The rich and the "sensitive" areas show heaviest deposits of glycogen. Note quite extensive involvement of entire thickness of cerebral cortex both in front of and behind the site of trauma, which is itself necrotic and completely devoid of glycogen granules. Dimedone-PAS, ×3.4. (C) Same conditions as in Fig. 6 A except that different levels of the brain are cut coronally to show the magnitude of posterolateral extension of the glycogen accumulation (dark areas). The control side is not-ched. Dimedone-PAS-gallocyanin, ×3.5. (D) Hippocampus of a hemisphere coronally trans-ected as in Fig. 6 B. Mainly astrocytes and "neuropil", especially of the molecular layers, show considerable glycogen deposits. Dimedone-PAS, ×250. (E) Brain of a rat unilaterally incised parasagitally. Vital staining with Evan's blue was used to mark the oedema fluid, which here appears dark, and was found to be co-extensive with the glycogen deposits. Un-stained, ×4

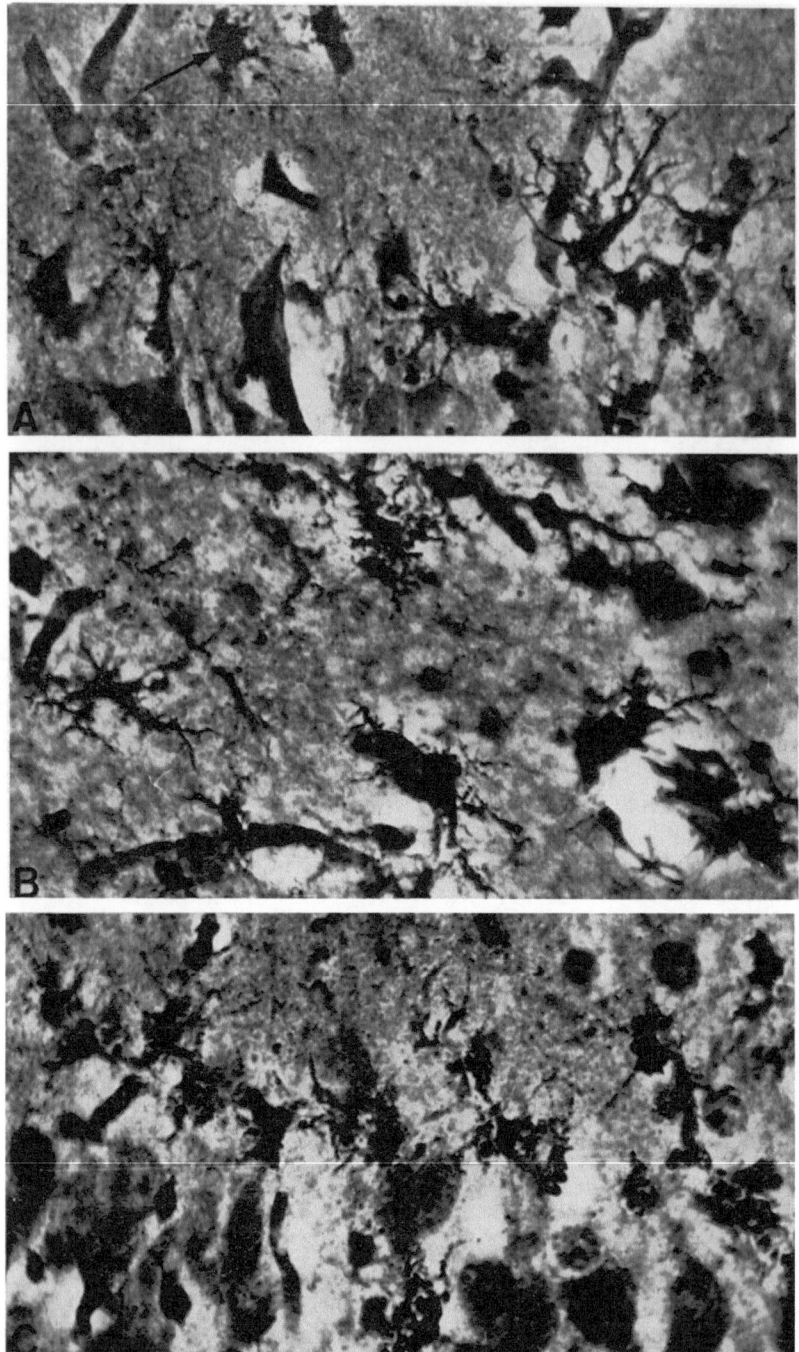

Fig. 7. (A) Pyriform cortex of a rat brain in which the olfactory bulb of one side was severed from the rest of the brain 48 hr previously. Probably all of the cells impregnated with silver are reactive oligodendrocytes in which both perikarya and processes are swollen. "Gliosomes" are prominent in some (arrow). Hortega's silver carbonate method for oligodendroglia, ×600. (B) Same animal and location as in Fig. 7A showing heavily impregnated and hypertrophied microglia; persistence of spiny processes indicates moderate reaction. Hortega's silver car-

Although our experiments on eye enucleation were unsuccessful in inducing glycogen deposits far from the insult, other observations were wade. In the injured partly shrunken contralateral optic tract, and allowing for possible factors vitiating the counts, increased numbers of oligodendroglia were noted, and fibrous astrocytes were seen hypertrophied and heavily impregnated with gold (Cajal's technique); in a similarly designed experiment Skoff and Price (1974) have noted an increase in the number of astrocytes. While noticeable after 7 days, these effects were most pronounced at 1–3 months, when microglial hypertrophy was obvious. Reactivity of these neuroglia was also noted in the stratum zonale and stratum griseum in the related anterior colliculus and in the lateral geniculate body as well. Only after 3 months was some glycogen seen in astrocytes and 'neuropil' in the degenerated shrunken parts of the optic chiasm. Apart from the changes in glycogen, these findings corroborate the autoradiographic and histologic findings of Altman and Das (1964), but not those of Chase (1943) who did not record any changes in the optic chiasm, optic tract or external geniculate body. It is interesting also that Dunkerley and Duncan (1969) did not see similar changes to ours in rat pyramidal fibers undergoing Wallerian degeneration, while Joseph (1954), working on the dorsal columns of the rabbit spinal cord, did. Furthermore, although Fuentes and Marty (1970) noted oligodendrogliosis in the auditory cortex upon destruction of the medial geniculate body they did not mention an increase in glycogen content. The reasons for these discrepancies elude us.

Oligodendroglial proliferation in indirectly injured optic chiasm and tract confirms the autoradiographic findings of Skoff and Vaughn (1971) and is of interest because it is an early event in demyelination and a response to direct injury of brain (Ibrahim et al., 1974).

It seems from the foregoing that the appearance of glycogen at long distances from the site of injury within only 1–2 days post-operatively can not be explained on the basis of neuronal degeneration, but neuroglial proliferation probably can; the work of Sjöstrand (1966a, b) on the deafferented rabbit hypoglossal nucleus confirms this. Involvement of a specific blood vessel and its area of distribution can not be implicated either (see Fig. 6B). On the other hand, the almost coextensive distribution of dye and glycogen in several experiments speaks strongly in favour of membrane permeability curtailment, obvious as oedema, in the causation of glycogen increase. Nevertheless, widespread arteriolar spasm, both reflexly and through possible release of 5-HT, could account for some, but not all, of the features of the glycogen distribution (see Irradiation and later discussion).

Glycogen accumulation in polymorphonuclear leucocytes outside the vascular boundaries has been observed previously by Marinesco (1928) and Friede (1954). It, also may be attributed to a maintained low grade hypoxic state as the cells leave the well-oxygenated confines of the blood vessels.

Our studies of enzymic changes confirmed the findings of Shimizu and Hamuro (1958), Ibrahim et al. (1968) and Farkas-Bargeton et al. (1972) concerning phosphorylase activity; as in irradiation, any cellular element that showed increase in glycogen also showed increase in phosphorylase activity (Figs. 8A and 9).

bonate method for microglia, ×600. (C) Same animal and location as in Fig. 7A showing hypertrophied and swollen protoplasmic astrocytes. Various size granules probably represent accumulations of glycogen. Cajal's gold-sublimate technique, ×600

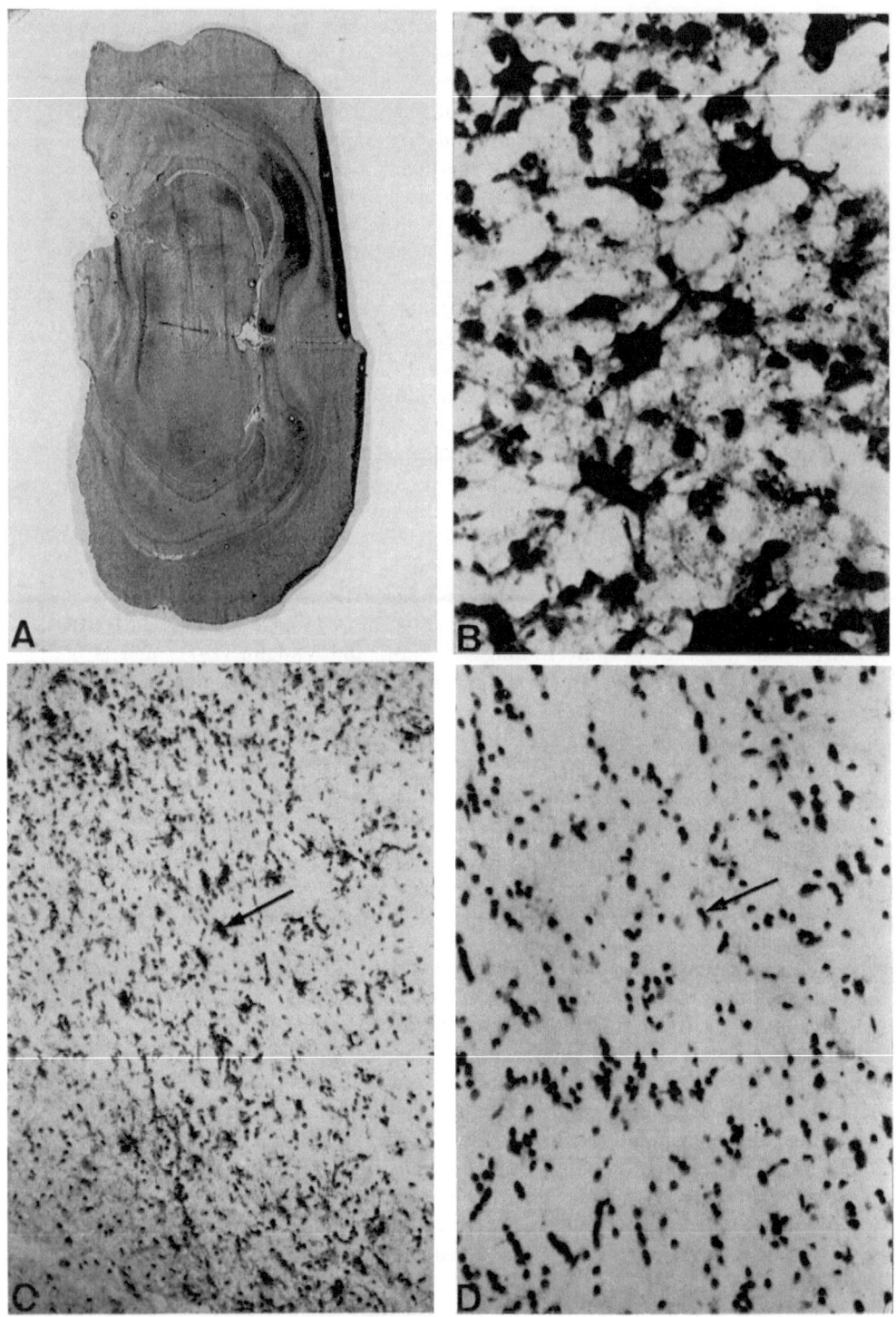

Fig. 8. (A) Cryostat section of a rat brain stabbed coronally just anterior to the level of the section 24 hr prior to sacrifice. Total phosphorylase activity is increased on the side of the stab (above) especially in the hippocampal formation, thalamus and inner cortex. Dilute

Oedematous white matter, when devoid of glycogen, showed greatly diminished activity (Fig. 8A). During the first hours after trauma there was a slight diminution of the activity of phosphorylase, phosphorylase + branching enzyme, as well glycogen synthetase, in the transition zone; the activity of hexokinase, which might reflect glucose entry, and of G-3-PD, a representative of the glycolytic pathway, was unchanged. Thereafter, activity of phosphorylase and phosphorylase + branching enzyme began to recover and to increase above normal by 6–8 hrs. One day later, glycogen synthetase was still diminished both in the necrotic and in the transition zones of the lesions while G-3-PD was diminished in the necrotic zone only. All enzymes, except apparently glycogen synthetase, then became hyperactive in the transition zone where glycogen had accumulated. By 3–5 days, all of these enzymes were still hyperactive (Fig. 8B) and glycogen synthetase had increased considerably around the lesion (Fig. 8C), where large amounts of glycogen still persisted. Reactions were always more prominent in grey than in white matter. Both astrocytes and "neuropil", and to a lesser extent oligodendroglia, showed the increased enzymic activities (Fig. 9A and B). Activated microglia (gitter cells) that had appeared by 3–5 days contained no glycogen and, of all the enzymes tested, only that of G-3-PD.

These enzymic changes suggest that direct trauma, which damages membrane permeability and compromises blood and oxygen supply and metabolic activity (Khan *et al.*, 1974), causes glycogen increase in "vulnerable" areas through a transient diminution in glycolysis in much the same way as envisaged for ionizing radiation and ischaemia (see pp. 44 & 62). The reason for the delay in increase in glycogen synthetase till after glycogen appeared is probably the same as discussed earlier. A *primary* increase in glycogen synthesis does not seem tenable here.

Hypoxia and Ischaemia

It is well known that hypoxia, anoxia or ischaemia, as such, cause a diminution or loss of glycogen. On the other hand, during recovery from these, an increase in CNS glycogen occurs (Hager, 1966; Hirano *et al.*, 1967; Bakay and Lee, 1968; Mossakowski *et al.*, 1968; Ibrahim *et al.*, 1968, 1970b; Rivera *et al.*, 1970; Śmialek *et al.*, 1971; Pronaszko-Kurczyńska *et al.*, 1971; Ibrahim, 1972; Long *et al.*, 1972; Schneider and Dralle, 1973; Śmialek *et al.*, 1973; Ito *et al.*, 1974). The various forms of hypoxia and ischaemia include that induced by cyanide intoxication (Hirano *et al.*, 1967; Ibrahim *et al.*, 1968, 1970b), carbon monoxide intoxication (Śmialek *et al.*, 1973), repeated exposure to nitrogen (Hager, 1966), exposure to low atmospheric pressure and oxygen tension (Bakay, 1965; Bakay and Lee, 1968), total asphyxia (Mossakowski *et al.*, 1968; Rivera *et al.*, 1970), combined hypoxia and ischaemia (Ibrahim *et al.*, 1968, 1970b; Pronaszko-

Gram's iodine, ×5.3. (B) Cryostat section of a rat brain stabbed 5 days previously. The cerebral cortex-close to the site of injury-shows hypertrophied, proliferated and enzymically hyperactive astrocytes and oligodendrocytes. Hexokinase, ×600. (C) Adjacent section to that of Fig. 8B shows somewhat proliferated, but considerably hypertrophied, fibrous astrocytes of corpus callosum (arrow). Oligodendrocytes are similarly reactive. Glycogen synthetase. Dilute Gram's iodine, ×150. (D) Opposite (control) side of the section from which Fig. 8C was taken. Normal glycogen synthetase activity is not very obvious but is evident in some astrocytes (arrow). Dimedone-PAS-Hematoxylin, ×250

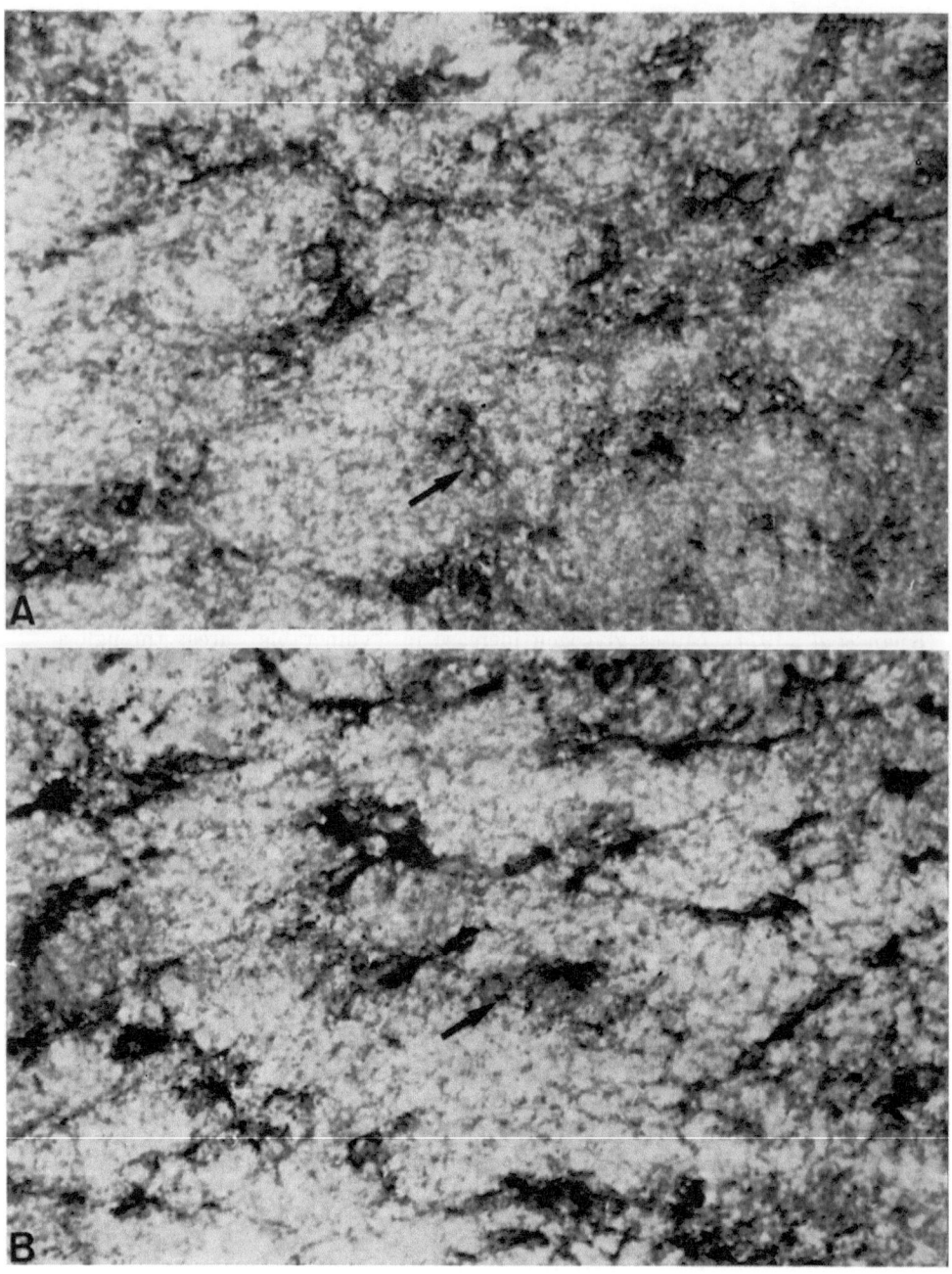

Fig. 9. (A) Phosphorylase activity in a cryostat-cut section of the normal (control) callosal angle of a rat brain directly traumatized (stab wound) 24 hr previously; arrow points to oligodendroglial activity. PAS, ×560. (B) Identical area on the stab side. Note enhanced activity in relation to the astrocytes; the status of the oligodendroglia (arrow) is difficult to distinguish from that of the control side. The "neuropil" is oedematous and activity in it is reduced. PAS, ×560

Kurczyńska et al., 1971; Śmialek et al., 1971) and ligation of the abdominal aorta (Long et al., 1972; Schneider and Dralle, 1973).

Several other studies have tackled various other aspects of induced hypoxia and ischaemia. For instance, Lindberg (1963) advanced the idea that the morphological changes which accompany hypoxaemia, such as brain oedema, selective ischaemic cell damage or complete softening are not immediately due to lack of oxygen and metabolic substrates but to intracellular acidosis—lactic acid accumulation. Such acidosis could develop only if the anoxia were stagnant and rapidly developing so that glucose is incompletely metabolized. Zeman (1963), who employed Levine's (1960) hypoxia-ischaemia model on monkeys and rats, found that in the early infarction stage all oxidative enzymes were decreased. During later reactive phases oxidative enzymic activity increased especially in proliferating astrocytes-increase in H^3-thymidine uptake. Spector (1961) and Plum et al., (1963) who employed light microscopy, and Brown and Brierley (1968, 1972) and McGee-Russell et al. (1970), who used electron microscopy in the study of anoxia, with and without ischaemia, as well as Arsénio-Nunes et al., (1973), who studied ischaemia alone, described the earliest event-neuronal swelling and microvacuolation-as due to swollen (oedematous) mitochondria and endoplasmic reticulum. Swollen astrocytic processes around such neurons, swollen capillary endothelium and pericytes and endothelial flaps (Arsénio-Nunes et al., 1973) were also seen. It is notable that McGee-Russell et al. (1970) found a simultaneous density of neuronal cytoplasm and an increase in neuronal ribosomal content indicating perhaps enhanced protein (enzyme) synthesis? In spite of the fact that some studies were extended to 24 hr postexposure no reference to glycogen was made. An interesting conclusion was a belief that hypoxia alone causes brain lesions by an ischaemic mechanism; the most vulnerable areas of brain were much the same as we have described (Ibrahim et al., 1970 b). We, (Ibrahim, 1972), had studied some aspects of this vulnerability by comparing the extent of damage in the different "sensitive" sites under various conditions, viz. hypoxia, ischaemia and combined ischaemia and hypoxia, and found that vulnerability, and hence sites of lesions, varied somewhat. We also noted the continued vulnerability of such sites to a relatively inocuous hypoxic episode after an apparently mild, fully-recoverable ischaemic insult. The vulnerability continued up to the time limit of the experiment, 6 days. Our conclusions, along with those of others, regarding regional susceptibilities will be discussed at the end.

It is of interest that chronic hypoxia (24 days in 10% oxygen, 90% nitrogen) gives a different pathological picture from that of acute hypoxia (Yu et al., 1972a, b). These authors, working on rat brain, found the swelling involved the Golgi apparatus as much as the other organelles in neurons. Again, glycogen was not mentioned either in relation to neurons or to swollen oligodendrocytes and astrocytes.

The studies in which workers have noted accumulation of glycogen have entailed varied methods of induction of hypoxia and ischaemia, varied animal species and varied age of animals, and have allowed animals to recover for periods longer than 12 hr. Generally, the glycogen appeared at the same cytological sites as described under irradiation and direct trauma, viz. astrocytic perivascular feet and perikarya and "neuropil" and, uncommonly, oligodendroglia. Only two studies described glycogen accumulation in neurons. One was the study by Long et al., (1972) on the spinal cord of the cat exposed to partial ischaemia produced by ligation of the abdominal aorta; the accumulated glycogen was seen in the astrocytes and large motor neurons in the anterior horns. The other was the study of carbon monoxide intoxication of Śmialek *et al.*, (1973) in which neuronal glycogen was in neurons of brain stem reticular formation and cranial nerve nuclei. Whereas generally glycogen started to increase appreciably at 6–8 hr post-exposure the neuronal accumulation of the study of Long *et al.* was seen as early as 1 hr and intraglial accumulation was at $1/_2$ hr; the carbon monoxide poisoning of Śmialek *et al.*, (1973) caused glycogen build-up by 1 hr. Thereafter, the accumulation increased to a maximum by about 24 hr in the ischaemia, and this is in uniformity with other studies in relation to neuroglia; glycogen maximum in the carbon monoxide study was much earlier, at 4 hr. It is probable that the identification of glycogen build-up was made possible only because the studies were by both light and electron microscopy and it is interesting that at neither level were other morphological changes seen. This, as noted above, is contrary to all other studies and can, perhaps be reconciled to the milder hypoxias.

Gross topographic distribution of the lesions has varied. Thus, Mossakowski *et al.*, (1968) and Rivera *et al.*, (1970), who exposed foetal monkeys delivered by Caesarian section to total anoxia—by asphyxia—for up to 14–16 min, found maximal damage in the thalamic ventrolateral nucleus, subthalamic nucleus, lateral geniculate body, inferior colliculus, vestibular nucleus, dentate nucleus and anterior horn of spinal chord; in white matter no lesions were seen but the most heavily myelinated areas contained sparse glycogen granules while those still undergoing myelination showed the heaviest deposits. On the other hand, the areas several workers, including ourselves, found most susceptible to milder anoxia, hypoxia, ischaemia and ischaemia-hypoxia in the rat and cat were the hippocampus (not dentate gyrus), the outer regions of the neocortex, parts of the amygdaloid area, deeper parts of the pyriform cortex, corpus striatum and parts of the thalamus (see Fig. 10) (Levine, 1960; Becker and Barron, 1961; McDonald and Spector, 1963; Lucas and Strangeways, 1963; Ibrahim *et al.*, 1970; Ibrahim, 1972b). This disagreement may reflect the variations in methodology, etc., mentioned above. The distribution of cyanide-induced lesions is unique in selectively including also large areas of white matter such as corpus callosum and callosal radiation (see Fig. 12) (Ferraro, 1933; Hurst, 1944; Hicks, 1950; Lumsden, 1950; Levine and Stypulkowski, 1959; Van Houten and Friede, 1961; Ibrahim *et al.*, 1963; Adams *et al.*, 1965; Ibrahim and Levine, 1967). Involvement of white matter was seen occasionally, however, in our hypoxic-ischaemic material. This similarity between hypoxic-ischaemic and cyanide lesions suggested to us that inhibition of cytochrome oxidase can not be the only cause of cyanide-induced lesions; an ischaemic element probably contributes as well (Levine and Klein, 1960; Ibrahim *et al.*, 1970b). This brings to mind the

Fig. 10. (A) Unilaterally ischaemic brain exposed 24 hr prior to sacrifice to unusually severe hypoxia. Glycogen is greatly increased in and around usual sites on both sides. Note lamination in the cerebral cortex due to variation in degree of damage. Layer II (and may be III) shows intense reaction in one part where there is moderate damage while in immediately adjacent severely damaged area the same layer is devoid of deposits. The amygdaloid complex on the ischaemic side (asterisk) contains less glycogen than that on the opposite side. Paraffin section. PAS, ×6. (B) Increased phosphorylase activity in usual sites of a rat brain exposed 6 hr prior to sacrifice to hypoxic hypoxia (lower); above is a normal control brain.

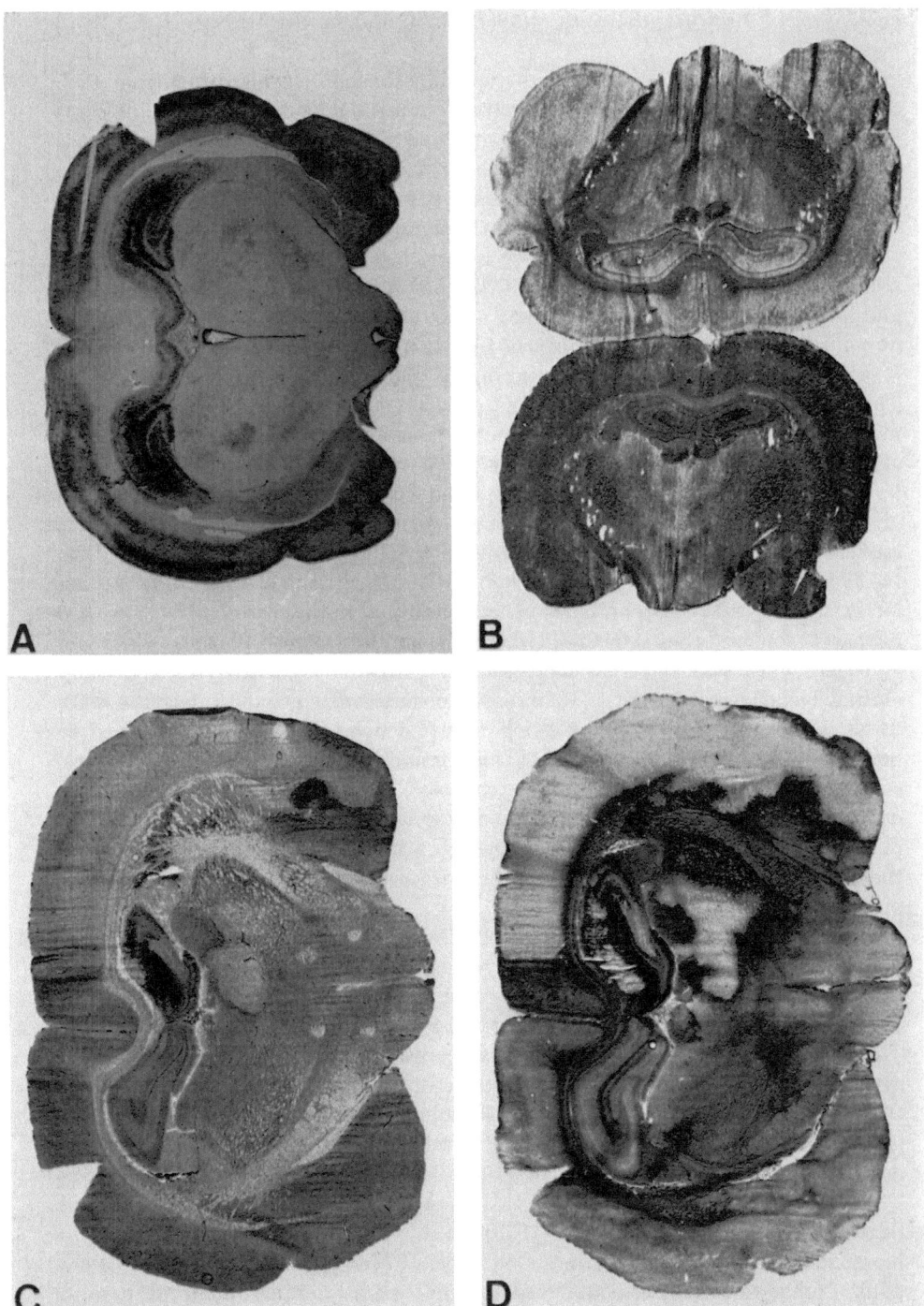

Dilute Gram's iodine, ×3.8. (C) Cryostat section of an ischaemic-hypoxic rat brain, 24 hr after the hypoxic episode, stained for glycogen. Compare with Fig. 10D. PAS, ×5.6. (D) Adjacent cryostat section to that shown in Fig. 10C demonstrating phosphorylase activity. The identical distribution of the enhanced polysaccharide and its hydrolytic enzyme is obvious. Dilute Gram's iodine, ×5.6

conclusion of Brown and Brierley (1968, 1972) and McGee-Russell et al., (1970) (see p. 55).

Although anoxic, ischaemic and hypoxic-ischaemic lesions differ from each other somewhat it is still the "sensitive" areas that suffer most in all cases (Ibrahim, 1972). We found the glycogen excesses located in and around the "sensitive" areas, either spread throughout if damage was not severe, or at the periphery of a central necrotic zone if damage was severe (Fig. 10). It is of interest to note that these "sensitive" areas are the same as those involved in phenobarbital anesthesia, exposure to ionizing radiation and direct traumatic damage (Ibrahim et al., 1970a, b; Ibrahim, 1972) (compare Figs, 5A, B, 6C, 8A, 10A, C and D). Furthermore, these "sensitive" areas do not only show increased glycogen on mild derangement but are "also the first to undergo necrosis when the damage is severe" (Ibrahim et al., 1970b; Ibrahim, 1972) (compare Fig. 10A with C and D). The areas adjacent to these sensitive ones are the areas that normally show most glycogen and are generally the most resistant, invariably enhancing their glycogen upon mild to moderate damage.

Relatively few authors have attempted histochemical correlates between glycogen and its related enzymes of metabolism, as compared with those who studied biochemical correlates (Mossakowski et al., 1968a, b; Ibrahim et al., 1968, 1970a; Rivera et al., 1970; Śmialek et al., 1971, 1973; Long et al., 1972; Ibrahim, 1972). Mossakowski et al. and Rivera et al. found that in those areas of asphyxiated neonatal monkey brain showing glycogen accumulation both phosphorylase and glycogen synthetase activities increased gradually in the astrocytes, especially around blood vessels, from 1–12 hr postexposure and started to decrease after 24 hr; glycogen reached almost twice control values by 12 hr and returned to normal by 48 hr. Mossakowski et al. also found that oxidoreductive enzymes, succinate dehydrogenase, cytochrome oxidase, NADH-dehydrogenase and lactate dehydrogenase decreased and remained low until 12 hr and then started to recover; glucose-6-phosphate dehydrogenase activity was decreased throughout the period of observation. All enzymic activity was reduced *within* the focal areas of damage.

Long et al., working on the partially-ischaemic cat spinal cord, noted an increase in both phosphorylase and glycogen synthetase. The former increased concurrently with the glycogen whereas the latter increased before the glycogen did; the glycogen buildup reached maximum by 24 hr and disappeared by 10 days. They suggested that the increased glycogen was due to the enhanced glycogen synthetase which, in turn, was presumably stimulated by an accumulated G-6-P; they did not suggest a source for this G-6-P. Furthermore, regarding phosphorylase increase, they suggested "that glycogen itself is a factor, which stimulates the activity of this enzyme (Nelson et al., 1968)".

Śmialek et al. (1971) used 28 day old Wistar rats subjected to bilateral carotid ligation, whereas Śmialek et al., (1973) used Wistar rats subjected to carbon monoxide poisoning. We (Ibrahim et al., 1968, 1970a; Ibrahim, 1972) used young adult Sprague-Dawley rats subjected to bilateral, as well as unilateral, carotid ligation, severe hypoxic hypoxia, combined hypoxic hypoxia with unilateral carotid ligation, and histotoxic (cyanide) hypoxia. Śmialek et al., (1971) noted that both active and total phosphorylase were increased from 12 hr, reached maximum by 72 hr and returned to normal by 120 hr. Glycogen synthetase activity showed a transient increase between 12 and 48 hr and returned to normal levels by 72 hr. On the other hand, Śmialek *et al.*, (1973) noted biochemically maximal glycogen synthetase activity at only 2 hr; thereafter both the enzyme and the glycogen—after 4 hr—gradually decreased to normal values by 120 hr. Because the maximal glycogen synthetase seemed to coincide with, or even precede, the greatest increment in glycogen they believed it probable that the increase in the enzyme was responsible for the glycogen build-up. To account for the increase in enzymic activities they (1971) suspected that glycogen synthetase was enhanced by an increase in the –SH pool and/or an increase in G-6-P; the enhanced phosphorylase may have been due to a rise in catecholamine, with consequent stimulation of the adenyl cyclase—cAMP—phosphorylase kinase system, as a result of the stress of the operative procedure.

The rat brains in our experiments contained abnormally large amounts of glycogen in all models except the unilateral ischaemic; the glycogen was seen unequivocally at 6–8 hr (Figs. 10–12). An increase in phosphorylase and phosphorylase + branching enzyme was also noted early, at 1 hr, after an initial transient period of reduction below normal. This phosphorylase increase was at the same site and in the same cells as the glycogen increase (Figs. 10C, D, 11A, B, C and 12D). Glycogen synthetase activity was slightly increased at all sites of phosphorylase hyperactivity. As would be predicted, activity of cytochrome oxidase and succinate and lactate dehydrogenases was initially decreased only at sites of more severe damage and remained low as necrosis set in. An increase at the edges of such areas did develop at 1 day or so but a more generalized increase was also noted in the non-necrotic areas of the brains including that of hexokinase (Fig. 11D) and 6-phosphogluconate dehydrogenase (see Zeman, 1963). Biochemical estimates of total phosphorylase in brains 16–24 hr after bilateral common carotid ligation showed that it increased by 129–179% (Ibrahim *et al.*, 1970b).

In their analysis of the mechanism(s) of glycogen accumulation Mossakowski and his co-workers have regarded damage to the neuron as central. They cited reduced glycogen utilization in the anoxic-ischaemic rat brain (Atkinson and Spector, 1964) and argued that neurons, being "the main consumers of glycogen", would suffer first and most severely. Puzzling to them was the accumulation of glycogen in neuroglia, especially astrocytes, rather than in neurons, as they would have expected. Since the role of astrocytes in fluid and glucose transport is well established, these authors found it "conceivable to envisage a situation in which damaged neurons are incapacitated to utilize properly the glucose which then begins to pile up in astrocytes and is converted, at the same time, into glycogen for storage". In support of this they presented their observation of increased phosphorylase and glycogen synthetase activities early post exposure. They suggested that the same explanation could be applied to glycogen accumulation in astrocytes "in the vicinity of brain tumors, stab wounds and particularly as effect of irradiation". The finding of increased glycogen in astrocytes—and oligodendrocytes—of myelinating white matter, which are unrelated to neurons, was interpreted as a reflection of the high energy demand of those areas undergoing myelination. In their carbon monoxide study, on the other hand, Śmialek *et al.*, (1973) attributed the glycogen build-up to the increase in activity of glycogen synthetase, i.e. directly increased synthesis in neurons, as well as astrocytes, etc. They could not account for the increased glycogen synthetase itself.

During an episode of hypoxic hypoxia or ischaemia of CNS or PNS, phosphocreatine, glycogen, glucose, G-6-P, fructose-6-phosphate and ATP decrease, while

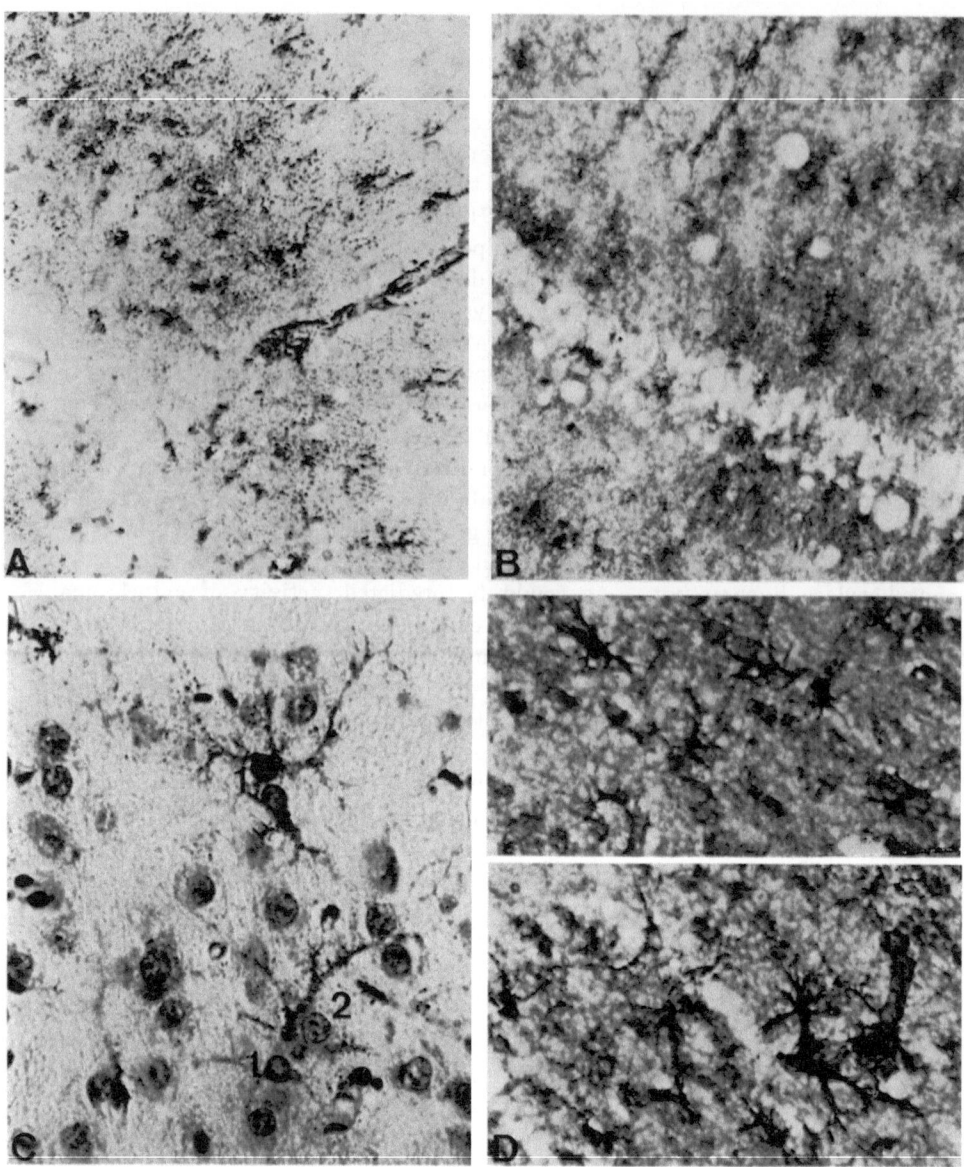

Fig. 11. (A) Hippocampus of the ischaemic-hypoxic side of a rat brain 24 hr after hypoxia.
Glycogen deposits are obvious in the "neuropil" and astrocytes of the molecular layers and
outline a blood vessel. Dimedone-PAS, ×210. (B) Similar area to that in Fig. 11A showing
increased phosphorylase activity in astrocytes and around blood vessels. Dilute Gram's
iodine, ×210. (C) Corpus striatum of a hypoxic-ischaemic rat brain 24 hr. after hypoxia. This
area which is adjacent to a severely damaged one (not shown) contains swollen glycogen-laden
oligodendrocytes (1) and an astrocyte (2). Dimedone-PAS gallocyanin, ×350. (D) Cerebral
cortex of a hypoxic-ischaemic rat brain 48 hr after hypoxia showing activity of hexokinase.
Enlarged and hyperactive astrocytes and oligodendrocytes are prominent in areas adjoining
more severely damaged ones (not illustrated). ×370

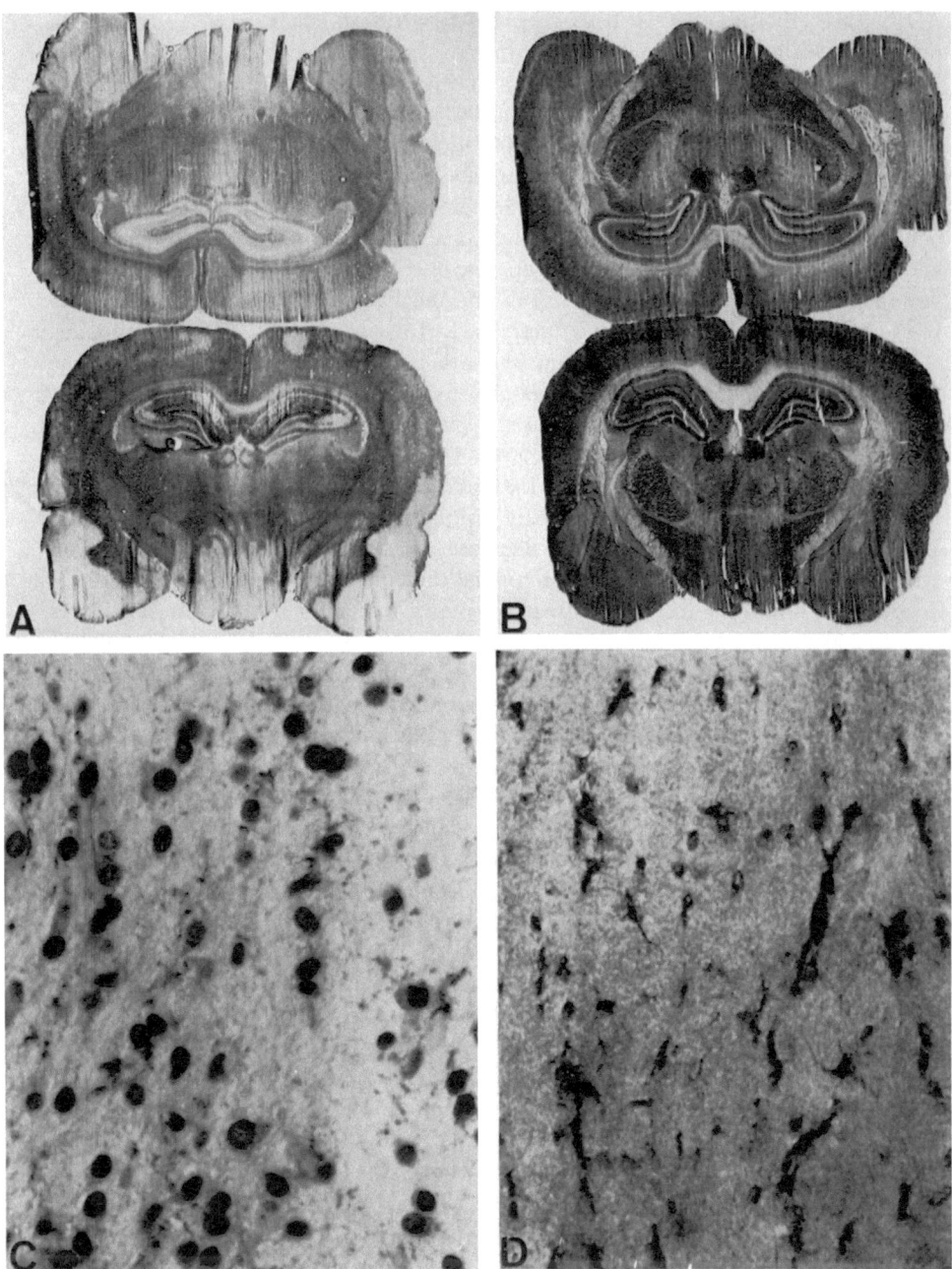

Fig. 12. (A) Cyanide-exposed rat brain (below), with a control, shows phosphorylase activity. Areas of severe damage are completely devoid of activity while the rest of the brain shows an increase. Dilute Gram's iodine, ×4. (B) Cyanide brain and its control (above) showing severe involvement of the corpus callosum only. The rest of the brain, but especially areas of grey matter, are enzymically hyperactive. Phosphorylase. Dilute Gram's iodine, ×4. (C) Callosal angle of a cyanide brain showing glycogen granules scattered in the "neuropil" rather than distinctly localised in neuroglial elements. Blood vessels are lightly outlined with granules. Dimedone-PAS-gallocyanin. ×510. (D) Corpus callosum of a normal brain showing activity of NADH-dehydrogenase. All neuroglial elements and vessel walls are seen. ×250

ADP, AMP, inorganic phosphate (Pi), fructose-1,6-diphosphate, α-glycerophosphate, lactate and acetyl coenzyme A increase, i.e. there is hyperactivity of the Embden-Meyerhof pathway; return to normal takes place at varying speeds (Albaum and Chinn, 1953; Lowry et al., 1964; Stewart et al., 1965; Stewart and Moonsammy, 1966; Gatfield et al., 1966; Schuberth et al., 1966; Maker et al., 1966; Folbergrová et al., 1970; Broniszewska-Ardlet and Jongkind, 1971; Duffy et al., 1972). In general, it should be remembred, however, that PNS can not behave like CNS and that ischaemic hypoxia differs from hypoxic hypoxia (or anoxia) in that the former entails hypoxia plus a deprivation of the tissues of metabolites, e.g. glucose, and a lack of the mechanism for removal of the end products of metabolic activity, e.g. lactic acid. However, because in every hypoxia there is also an element of ischaemia (see later), lactate accumulation was found to be actually higher in severe hypoxia (4% oxygen, 96% nitrogen) than in ischaemia of mouse brain (Broniszewska-Ardlet and Jongkind, 1971). These workers attributed the lactate accumulation partly to more economical glycolysis in the presence of hypoxia and also noted that phosphocreatine dropped to only 70% of normal,while in ischaemia it virtually disappeared within 3 min. Nevertheless, Duffy et al., (1972) did not record a decrease in ATP or creatine phosphate, but still found that during 30 min of hypoxia the metabolic rate of mouse brain decreased by 15% or more. Following recovery in air for 10 min brain glucose rose to 200% and there was an increase in G-6-P, creatine phosphate and citrate, while fructose-1,6-diphosphate diminished; lactate and pyruvate remained high. These authors interpreted the diminution in fructose-1,6-diphosphate and the increase in G-6-P as indicating a block at the phosphofructokinase level possibly due to inhibition by the increased creatine phosphate and citrate, i.e. there was effective diminution in anaerobic glycolysis. There was also an obvious malfunction of the citric acid cycle, as evidenced by the high pyruvate, which in turn kept the level of acetyl coenzyme A high and prevented a fall in citrate.

The overall picture then *during* hypoxia is one of hyperactivity of the Embden-Meyerhof pathway and possibly also defective citric acid cycle; during recovery both the pathway and the cycle are, at least for some time, more sluggish than normal. Also, any form of hypoxia damages the enzymic makeup of, and ion transport mechanisms across all membranes, plasma, nuclear, mitochondrial, etc. (Brown and Brierley, 1968, 1972; McGee-Russell et al., 1970 above) and recovery of these is slow. As mentioned earlier, such membrane damage leads to loss of intracellular K^+, increase in intracellular Na^+ and oedema, which further depress glycolysis (see p. 44). Furthermore, lactic acid accumulation, with its consequent drop in intracellular pH, may cause structural damage (Lindeberg, 1963) and, in itself, stimulate glycogen synthesis (Hassid et al., 1951).

Another factor already mentioned as operative in generalized irradiation is the hyperglycaemia which also accompanies generalized hypoxia, in contrast with localized (ischaemic) hypoxia. This was described by Thorn et al. (1959) but denied by Duffy et al., (1972). Nevertheless, as mentioned above, Duffy et al. recorded a 200% increase in brain glucose after 10 min of recovery in air; hyperglycaemia with consequent rise in brain glucose and glycogen has been discussed above. Furthermore, hypoxia is said to stimulate phosphorylation of glucose (Passonneau and Lowry, 1962) and, hence, to facilitate glycogen synthesis.

It seems therefore that glycogen build-up during recovery from all forms of hypoxia is effected through diminished glycolysis and consequent increased glycogenesis; in generalized hypoxia hyperglycaemia probably contributes significantly. Our finding of increased hexokinase activity could be interpreted to indicate heightened transport of glucose; Go *et al.*, (1974) have described an increase in facilitated diffusion from blood to brain of ischaemic gerbils and hypoxic rabbits. The increased 6-phosphogluconate dehydrogenase could reflect hyperactivity of the pentose shunt to compensate for the reduction in glycolysis (Ibrahim *et al.*, 1970b).

The enzyme mainly responsible for the synthesis of the excess glycogen is in all probability glycogen synthetase even though in our material, and in that of Śmialek *et al.*, (1971), obvious increases in this enzyme's activity appeared usually a little later than did the new glycogen and enhanced phosphorylase. However, Mossakowski and his group and Śmialek *et al.*, (1973) did note an increase in glycogen synthetase prior to that in glycogen. Also, the normal amount of this enzyme in brain is theoretically capable of synthesizing 12 times the amount of glycogen normally present (Breckenridge and Crawford, 1961) and hence an increase in synthesis need not perhaps always be accompanied by detectable increases in enzymic activity. Śmialek *et al.*, (1973) recorded glycogen increase before heightened glycogen synthetase at 0 hr after exposure to 60 min of carbon monoxide; later both increased as mentioned earlier. As indicated above G-6-P was found by several authors to be increased and the effect, at least theoretically, of this on both glycogen synthetase and phosphorylase has already been mentioned. It is of interest that Goldberg and O'Toole (1969) noted that anoxia (by decapitation) of rat brain caused a 3–4 fold rise in glycogen synthetase-I which suggested to them, "that a species of the I form of brain synthetase may provide a suppressive role rather than the facilitatory role recognized in other tissues." It has already been mentioned that these authors believe that glycogen control in brain is unique in that it appears to lack the requirement for D to I synthetase conversion.

The enzyme mainly responsible for breakdown of glycogen is phosphorylase. Paradoxically, it increased at about the same time as did the glycogen but after a very early decrease coincident with the well known glycogen loss of the "Pasteur effect" (Lowry *et al.*, 1964). The sequence of events envisaged by us (Ibrahim *et al.*, 1970b) is that within *seconds* of the onset of hypoxia, and while ATP levels are still normal (see Duffy *et al.*, 1972), inactive phosphorylase b is transformed to the active a form through activation of phosphorylase kinase by cAMP (Breckenridge and Norman, 1962); the activation could be, as Śmialek *et al.* (1971) envisage it, due to the rise of catecholamine as a result of the stress of the hypoxic procedure. The increase in phosphorylase a would be responsible for the "Pasteur effect". Soon, ATP level falls and AMP and Pi rise (see above) with consequent reduction in active phosphorylase for some minutes (see Ibrahim, 1968). During reoxygenation and recovery ATP synthesis is restored and so is phosphorylase activity which then even exceeds normal due to the increasing glycogen; this, as mentioned above, could be an adaptive mechanism to maintain the balance of the new structural-functional unit for more efficient utilization of the glycogen (Selinger and Schramm, 1963; Prasannan and Subrahmanyam, 1968b). Both the increased phosphorylase activity, as well as the excessive glycogen, are presumably maintained until full recovery of the metabolic machinery at which time the unit, with all its components, returns to normal.

This is only one possible explanation for maintained phosphorylase hyperactivity with glycogen excesses apparently unaffected by it. An alternative, or additional, explanation is based on the afore-mentioned dependence of phosphorylase activity on the physical characteristics of the glycogen. Glycogen, varying as it does in molecular weight, could under such abnormal conditions be not only excessive but also of such molecular size, e.g. large, and configuration that it would bind more of the enzyme and more strongly especially its active form (see p. 33 and Tata, 1964; Mršulja et al., 1968; Takeuchi, 1970).

The reason is not clear why glycogen accumulation has been described only in neuroglia in almost all studies, except that of Long et al. (1972) and Śmialek et al. (1973) in which neurons were also involved. Although Mossakowski et al. suggested that primary neuronal damage is responsible for this accumulation of neuroglial glycogen we can not agree with this for several reasons. Except for the isolated case of the directly traumatized rat cortical neurons, we did not detect an increase in glycogen or its enzymes, or in the oxidoreductive enzymes of neurons in areas showing glycogen accumulation. In areas of neuronal necrosis, all other cellular elements also showed necrosis, and glycogen was diminished or disappeared everywhere. In the glycogen-rich zones, maximal build-up was in astrocytes whereas perineuronal oligodendrocytes, which form a more clearly symbiotic unit with neurons (Friede and van Houten, 1962; Hydén 1962, 1967; Hamberger and Sjöstrand, 1966), rarely showed glycogen accumulation except in severe cases. Accumulation of glycogen in fibrous astrocytes and in oligodendrocytes of white matter also can not be accounted for on the basis of primary neuronal involvement. In addition, even in the case of the directly injured neurons mentioned above the injury had to be optimal and, furthermore, not all grisea involved showed glycogen accumulation, but only the special "sensitive areas". The reasons for this regional selectivity and involvement of neuroglia related to certain neurons only are not understood but will be discussed later.

Comment is perhaps needed regarding the cyanide-induced lesions, especially that cyanide intoxication is the only condition in which lesions could be confined to white matter (Fig. 12 A and B) (see above references). Both Hirano et al. (1967) and we (Ibrahim et al., 1968, 1970 b) noted glycogen accumulation in such damaged white matter some 24 hr postexposure. Using electron microscopy, Hirano et al. localized the glycogen in swollen glial cells with irregular nuclei and cytoplasm containing accumulations of organelles and engulfed material. They regarded the lesions as constituting primary damage affecting coursing axons with secondary involvement of adjacent neuroglia and myelin. No neuronal damage was observed. In our light microscopic study both astroglia and oligodendroglia, as well as "neuropil", were the main sites of the glycogen granules both in demyelinated white matter and around necrotic lesions of grey and white matter (Fig. 12C). Although white matter islands of the corpus striatum showed swollen, proliferated and PAS-positive oligodendrocytes and myelin pallor, glycogen was not evident.

As might have been expected, we noted at the sites of glycogen increase also intensified activity of phosphorylase (Fig. 12A and B) NADH- and NADPH-dehydrogenases (Fig. 13A and B; compare with control, Fig. 12D) and lactate and 6-phosphogluconate dehydrogenases (Fig. 13D; compare with control, Fig. 13C). This activity was located in reactive astrocytes and oligodendrocytes which were hypertrophied, swollen and increased in number. Necrotic and demyelinated areas naturally contained lower activities of all enzymes but the diminution of phosphorylase was always the most striking (Fig. 12A and B).

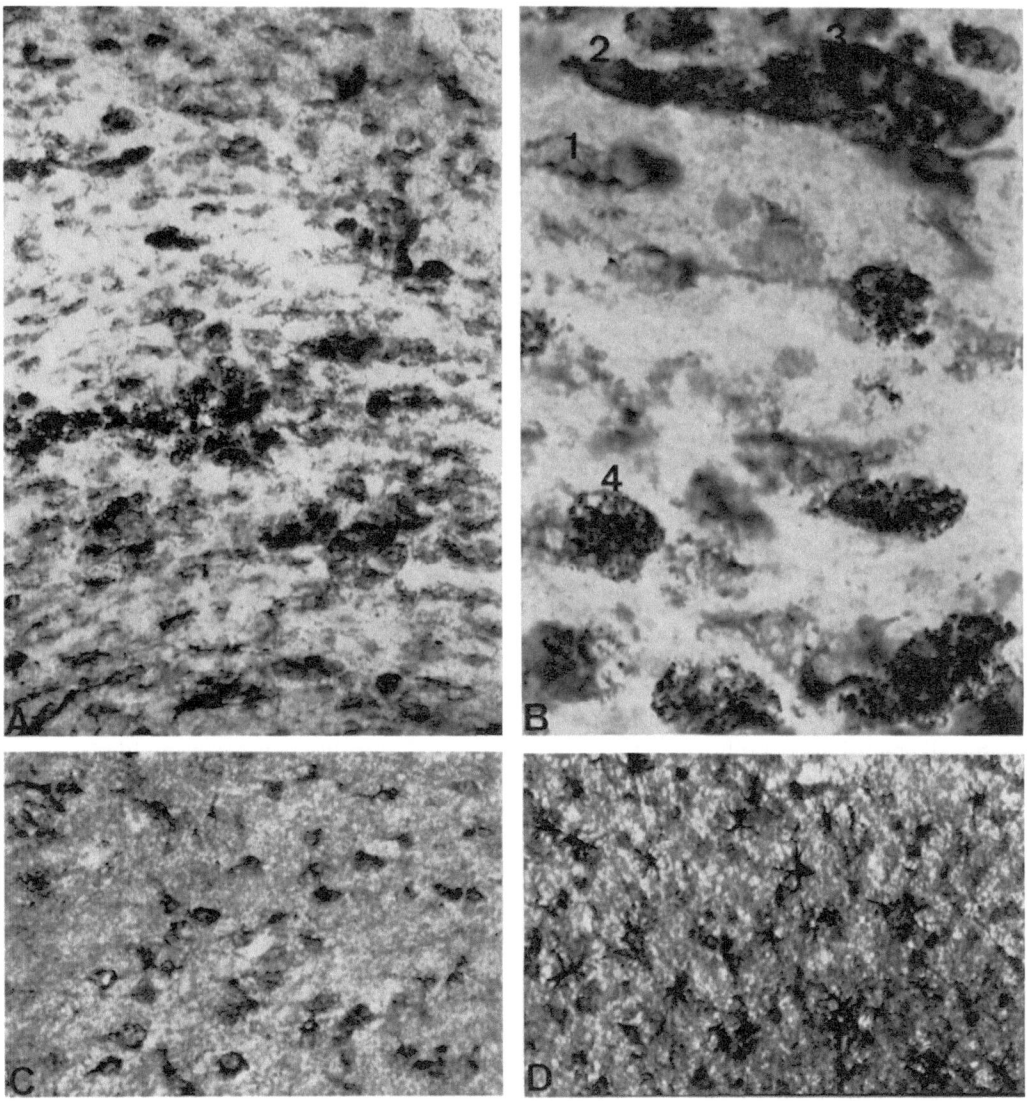

Fig. 13. (A) Corpus callosum of a rat brain exposed to HCN 4 days previously. Markedly proliferated, hypertrophied and swollen oligodendrocytes exhibit increased activity of NADH-dehydrogenase. Perivascular and interfascicular rows of oligodendrocytes are identifiable. Compare with control in Fig. 12D. ×250. (B) Higher magnification of part of Fig. 13A shows apparently normal (1) and perivascular, hypertrophied but not swollen oligodendrocytes (2), and an astrocyte (3). Considerably swollen oligodendrocytes with central nuclei and radiating cytoplasmic strands contain enlarged enzymically hyperactive "gliosomes" (4). NADH-dehydrogenase, ×625. (C) Normal rat parietal cerebral cortex shows activity of 6-phosphogluconate dehydrogenase. Neurons, and neuroglia the identity of which is difficult to determine, can be clearly seen. ×250. (D) Identical area and enzyme to that in Fig. 13C in a rat exposed 4 days previously to HCN. Enhanced activity is obvious in "neuropil" and neuroglia but not in neurons. ×250

Finally, the increase in glycogen noted by Mossakowski and his group, as well as by ourselves, in oligodendrocytes is of interest because of the observation of Haymaker *et al.*, (1972) that this is one of the earliest signs heralding delayed radiation necrosis in white matter. This pleads for a partially hypoxic aetiology for that condition due to abnormal vessels (see Haymaker, 1970; Ibrahim, 1974).

Hyperoxia

It is interesting that not only recovery from all forms of hypoxia but also breathing pure oxygen at 1 atmorpheric pressure for 2 hr increased the glycogen content of brain (young adult albino rat) from 3.38 to 4.35 μmoles glucosyl residues/g wet weight; there was a simultaneous drop in glucose and lactate (Gercken and Preuss, 1969). The capability of "storage of oxygen" by brain to "use for oxidative energy production", which has been suggested and which these authors had set out to test, was not indicated through this study.

7. General Discussion and Conclusions

Obviously, glycogen accumulation in the CNS occurs under a variety of conditions. Discussion of the possible mechanisms underlying this accumulation in the various conditions mentioned above indicates that a common mechanism for all conditions is probable. Also, it is obvious that the glycogen has a predilection to certain specific "sensitive" sites, a fact that could, perhaps, be used to advantage in clinical practice. These aspects need further discussion.

7.1. The Common Metabolic Derangement

Summarizing the various possible aetiological factors responsible for glycogen increase strongly suggests that the most important single common factor is a reduction in metabolic rate and glucose utilization. This, in turn, could be due to several mechanisms acting through depression of anaerobic glycolysis, with or without aerobic glycolysis, at various levels. In the case of exposure to cold or CNS depressants a *generalized* inhibition of metabolic activity was in fact shown. In the case of ionizing radiation, suppression of glycolysis would be achieved specifically through inhibition of the -SH dependent enzymes glyceraldehyde-3-phosphate dehydrogenase and ATPase, and inhibition of synthesis of coenzyme A and active acetate. Other mechanisms acting somewhat specifically through anaerobic glycolysis would be damage to the Na^+-pump and consequent loss of K^+ from cells by direct trauma, ionizing radiation and hypoxia, and the radiation-induced decrease in NAD. Naturally, the accompanying damage to membrane permeability would aggravate the effects on metabolism. It follows, therefore, that any cause of membrane damage, seen overtly as oedema, could induce a glycogen build-up; many of the human pathological conditions, accompanied by increased glycogen, can be viewed in this light.

The consequence in all cases is a rise in intracellular glucose levels. In the presence of a normally functioning glycogen metabolic cycle, this glucose, unable to leave the cell, is stored in the form of glycogen. The normally 12 times optimal content of glycogen synthetase might reasonably be expected not to increase demonstrably in order to effect this enhanced synthesis. Nevertheless, the activity of this enzyme was found to be increased when insulin + glucose injection was used to increase intracellular glucose. It was also increased in recovering asphyxiated neonatal monkey brain and rat brain recuperating from carbon monoxide poisoning. Generally as well, it has been usually assumed that whenever G-6-P is increased this would automatically stimulate activity of this enzyme while inhibiting that of phosphorylase, both effects presumably leading to the same end, enhanced glycogen.

An important general contributing factor is the rise in intracellar glucose, secondary to hyperglycaemia, in the presence of a defective mechanism for handling this glucose. This situation obtains during ionizing radiation and generalized hypoxia.

Other minor factors that could contribute include those that might inhibit phosphorylase activity and/or stimulate glycogen synthetase activity. Such a situation is seen, at least theoretically, when intracellular glucose is augmented causing an increase in G-6-P. The rise in glucose itself, as mentioned above, could be secondary to hyperglycaemia, with or without increased permeability, or a facilitation of carrier mediated glucose transport as in the presence of CNS depressants or excess insulin. Increased glucose phosphorylation, as in the presence of hypoxia, would also cause an increase in G-6-P. Furthermore, any cause of diminution in the adenyl cyclase system, causing as it does a diminution in cAMP, would decrease phosphorylase and increase glycogen synthetase activity; this happens when monoamines of brain are decreased. Again a decrease in inorganic phosphate would decrease phosphorylase activity whereas an increase in lactate, and a decrease in pH, generally tend to stimulate glycogenesis.

Special conditions of mal-function causing glycogen build-up would include damage to mechanisms usually acting in unison with phosphorylase in the control of glycogenolysis. Pompe's disease glycogenic storage would belong to this category since here lysosomal α-glucosidase is lacking. Other conditions would include Wallerian and retrograde degeneration where obviously decreased metabolic activity occurs but without many of the more drastic changes mentioned above

7.2. The "Vulnerable or Specific" Sites

Comparison of the sites normally rich in glycogen with those showing increased glycogen after exposure to moderate doses of ionizing radiation indicates that they are more or less identical, i.e. the excess glycogen could be regarded as representing an exaggeration of the normal state. When the radiation dose is quite large, but non-necrotic or rapidly lethal (see Haymaker *et al.*, 1972), glycogen appears in the poor areas adjacent to these sites. Exposure to some form of mild hypoxia will do the same, but if the hypoxic episode is more severe necrosis and loss of glycogen will take place primarily in the poor areas. Exaggeration of the rich sites will also occur; the rich sites, exemplified by the dentate gyrus, are the most resistant. Phosphorylase activity behaves similarly. Response to direct trauma follows the same pattern but, of course, depends on the "sensitivity" of the area and its distance from the site of trauma, i.e. severity.

Although these generalized statements probably have some credibility, as mentioned earlier, there are some differences in the way the "sensitive" sites respond to the different types of insult. This probably reflects the reason(s) for the sensitivity of a given site (pathoclisis) in the first place. These, according to Kety, (1963) are several and include the oxygen tension in arterial blood, perfusion rate and blood pressure, rate of oxygen utilization, available metabolic pathways and their susceptibility to hypoxia, length of capillary, intercapillary distance and capillary configuration, viz. "blood supply". The presence of energy reserves, principally glycogen, must also be important, and it is perhaps logical to assume that areas of the CNS apparently rich in it need this high content as an added protective mechanism. Foetal and neonatal heart survival under conditions of anoxia "is directly related to the pre-anoxic level of glycogen" (Dawes, 1963). It follows as well that glycogen increase as a response to insult of whatever type could logically be regarded as an increase in this energy reserve. It can also be argued that an increase in reserve means an anticipation of further damage. It is not surprising therefore that the glycogen-poor areas that show increases with mild or moderate damage are the ones to lose glycogen and show necrosis when the damage is more severe; normally rich areas become even richer and are spared to the last.

It is generally held "that normal glycogen levels are inversely related to the blood supply" (Folbergrová et al., 1970), i.e., the supply of oxygen, glucose and other nutrients, and the drainadge of metabolic end products. If therefore there is hypoxic, or anaemic, hypoxia (e.g. haemorrhage) mainly the oxygen delivery suffers, while if ischaemia occurs not only is the oxygen supply curtailed but so also is the supply of nutrients, and metabolites, such as lactate, are allowed to accumulate usually causing a drop in local pH and further aggravating matters (Dawes, 1963). However, when hypoxia is maintained capillaries first dilate but later show blood stasis, i.e. there is then an element of ischaemia as well (Meyer, 1963) and lactate accumulates. Also, Chiang et al. (1968), using the rabbit, and Arsénio-Nunes et al. (1973), using the cat, have shown that carotid ligation causes considerable encroachment on the capillary lumen through swelling of endothelium, creation of endothelial flaps, and perivascular glia; Hills (1964) reported lasting endothelial swelling in the rat on ischaemia-hypoxia. Such encroachement could perhaps progress to permanent occlusion in some parts (Ames et al., 1968). Furthermore, Crowell and Olsson (1972) found that temporary or sustained clamping of the middle cerebral artery of the monkey caused impairment of the filling of the microvasculature (see also Arsénio-Nunes et al., 1973; Ito et al., 1974); if there was hypotension during the occlusion, total non-filling of the microvasculature resulted. Even direct trauma of a monkey cerebral artery can cause generalized vasospasm in its branches lasting approximately 4 hr (Simeone et al., 1968); this, incidentally, could perhaps account for part of the more limited form of distribution of the neuroglial and glycogen changes described under "Direct trauma".

Because of the multiplicity of the factors determining the "sensitivity" of certain sites it becomes understandable why different causative agents can still affect predominently the same sites, with only little variation in the pattern. However, under certain conditions areas not usually regarded as "sensitive" may be affected, and sometimes almost selectively, e.g. white matter of callosal angles in some ischaemic-hypoxic and cyanide-induced lesions. This could perhaps reflect the reportedly high metabolic rate (see Folbergrová *et al.*, 1970) but poor blood supply of these white areas, which may make them more sensitive to ischaemia rather than to hypoxia.

Two further factors could be visualized as contributing to the "sensitivity" of certain areas of the CNS. The first is the presence, or absence, of collateral circulation. It is well known that collateral circulation in CNS is rather poor but it does exist, especially through leptomeningeal vessels (Crowell *et al.*, 1971; Rosenblum, 1974), and can account for the limited damage caused by middle cerebral artery occlusion (Meyer, 1958; Meyer and Portnoy, 1958; Crowell *et al.*, 1970); work on monkeys by Crowell *et al.* (1970) even lead them to suggest that embolectomy may be of use if done within 4 hr on humans. The second factor could be the presence of potentially active vasoactive substances such as 5-HT. This substance, as pointed out by Ibrahim (1972), is copious in certain of the "sensitive" areas such as some of those of the rhinencephalon (Passonen *et al.*, 1957; Samson, 1964). As pointed out earlier, it is possible that as a response to a noxious stimulus a sudden substantial release from its binding sites of such a substance could cause a vicious circle of vasospasm, haemostasis, increased membrane and vascular permeability, and oedema thus aggravating the condition (see Spector and Willoughby, 1957; Raynor *et al.*, 1961; Karlsberg *et al.*, 1962; Paasonen, 1965; Ibrahim, 1972; Welch *et al.*, 1973; Allen *et al.*, 1974; Wurtzman and Zervas, 1974).

Acknowledgments

I would like to thank Dr. Enid Pascoe of the Biology Department, and Dr. Usama Khalidi of the Biochemistry Department, American University of Beirut for their valuable suggestions and comments. I also wish to thank Mr. D. Koshayan for his technical assistance, Miss Shaké Mekhitarian for her secretarial work, Mr. H. Chohmelian for producing some of the photographs and Mr. A. Chalabian for drawing Fig. 1. Figs. 2C, D, E and 3D, E, F and 4C, D and 10B, C, D are reproduced by permission of the Editor-in-Chief, Journal of Neurological Sciences. Figs. 2A and 5A are reproduced by permission of Academic Press Inc. Fig. 10A is reproduced by permission of the Editor-in-Chief, American Journal of Pathology. Figs. 6A and B are reproduced by permission of S. Karger, Basel.

8. Summary

Although the glycogen content of the CNS is relatively small its function as an energy reserve is significant, and its turnover is considerable. Both glycogen and its related enzymes of metabolism—phosphorylase, branching enzyme and glycogen synthetase—are composed of various subunits and forms, most of which are histochemically distinguishable in the normal mammalian CNS. They have an essentially similar distribution, a fact that may reflect certain metabolic needs and inherent susceptibilities. They also undergo similar alterations as part of normal physiologic activity, as a result of exposure to certain physical or chemical stimuli or as a consequence of direct or indirect damage by, e.g. ionizing radiation, various forms and combinations of hypoxia and direct or indirect mechanical injury; the glycogen content is also increased in several human pathological states. When the stimulus is mild, and the response reversible, the glycogen content is temporarily enhanced within and around the sites that normally contain most glycogen. Activity of phosphorylase and glycogen synthetase usually undergo parallel increases then; the status of the branching enzyme is difficult to determine. Under these circumstances enzymes of the Embden-Meyerhof pathway, and some oxidoreductive enzymes, show less pronounced alterations. More noxious stimuli cause loss of glycogen and all enzymatic activity within necrotic foci and enhanced glycogen and enzymatic activity around such foci. The enzyme to show earliest, and most pronounced, reaction is phosphorylase; this distinguishes this enzyme as the most sensitive histochemical parameter of damage.

The parallel increases in glycogen and its enzymes probably reflect the attaintment of new levels of dependence on the glycogen-enzyme structural-functional unit for the metabolic demands. This dependence, in turn, can be considered to reflect a nonspecific defensive reaction to injury which may be anticipating further damage and/or acting as a temporary emergency mechanism; all changes short of the lethal are eventually reversible.

It is felt that the ultimate mechanism underlying glycogen increase under most conditions is basically the same; diminished glucose utilization through inhibited anaerobic metabolism, with or without inhibited aerobic metabolism, is probably the direct cause of the glycogen increase. Any accompanying hyperglycaemia would necessarily contribute by inducing an increase in glycogen synthesis. Increased glycogen synthetase activity, even though not necessarily demonstrable histochemically, effects the neoglycogenesis, and could be stimulated by heightened levels of glucose-6-phosphate and/or changes in nucleotide levels. Increased phosphorylase activity is probably due to more than one factor including changes in nucleotide levels, monoamine content and metabolic rate.

The sites adjacent to those normally showing largest glycogen content are revealed as the most vulnerable or susceptible to injury; the sites richest in glycogen are essentially the least susceptible. It is felt that the normally larger content of glycogen and its enzymes in certain sites must be an innate protective mechanism participating in a delicately balanced system in which an inherently labile blood supply, and/or a high content of potentially vasoactive substance, e.g. 5-HT, is reinforced by other defenses.

References

Adams, C.W.M., Ibrahim, M.Z.M., Leibowitz, S.: Demyelination. In: C.W. M. Adams (Ed.), p. 437 Neurohistochemistry. Amsterdam: Elsevier 1965

Albaum, H. G., Chinn, H.I.: Brain metabolism during acclimatization to high altitude: Amer. J. Physiol., **174**, 141–145 (1953)

Albrecht, W.: Erhöhung der Glykogen-Konzentration im Gehirn und das Verhalten verschiedener Fermente in Gehirn und Darm der Maus nach Reserpin (Serpasil), Klin. Wschr. **35**, 588–590 (1957)

Allen, G.S., Gold, L.H.A., Chou, S.N., French, L.A.: Cerebral arterial spasm, Part 3: *In vivo* intracisternal production of spasm by serotonin and blood and its reversal by phenoxybenzamine. J. Neurosurg. **40**, 451–458 (1974)

Altman, J., Das, G.D.: Autoradiographic and histological investigation of changes in the visual system of rats after unilateral enucleation. Anat. Rec. **148**, 535–545 (1964)

Ames, III, A., Wright, R.L., Kowada, M., Thurston, J.M., Majno, G.: Cerebral ischaemia, Part 2 (The no-reflow phenomenon). Amer. J. Path. **52**, 437–454 (1968)

Ammon, H.P.T., Estler, C.-J., Heim, F.: Der Einfluß von Äthylalkohol auf den Kohlen-hydrat- und Energiestoffwechsel des Gehirns weißer Mäuse, Arch. int. Pharmacodyn. Ther. **154**, 108–121 (1965)

Appleman, M.M., Krebs, E.G., Fischer, E.H.: Purification and properties of inactive liver phosphoryase. Bio-Chemistry (Wash.) **5**, 2101–2107 (1966)

Arsénio-Nunes, M.L., Hossmann, K.A., Farkas-Bargeton, E.: Ultrastructural and histo-chemical investigation of the cerebral cortex of cat during and after ischaemia. Acta neuropathol. (Berl.) **26**, 329–344 (1973)

Ashford, C.A., Dixon, K.C.: The effect of potassium on the glucolysis of brain tissue with reference to the Pasteur effect. Biochem. J. **29**, 157–168 (1935)

Atkinson, J.N.C., Spector, R.G.: Metabolism of glucose in anoxic-ischaemic rat brain. Brit. J. exp. Pathol. **45**, 393–397 (1964)

Bakay, L.: The movement of electrolytes in different types of cerebral edema. Prog. Brain Res. **15**, 155–183 (1965)

Bakay, L., Lee, J.C.: The effect of acute hypoxia and hypercapnia on the ultrastructure of the central nervous system, Brain, **91**, 697–706 (1968)

Barron, K.D., Doolin, P.F.: Ultrastructural observations on retrograde atrophy of lateral geniculate body. II. The environs of the neuronal soma, J. Neuropathol. exp. Neurol., **27**, 401–420 (1968)

Barron, K.D., Means, E.D., Larsen, E.: Ultrastructure of retrograde degeneration in the thalamus of rat. 1. Neuronal somata and dendrites. J. Neuropathol. exp. Neurol. **32**, 218–244 (1973)

Becker, N.H., Barron, K.D.: The cytochemistry of anoxic-ischaemic encephalopathy in rats, Part 1 (Alterations in neuronal lysosomes identified by acid phosphatase activity), Amer. J. Path., **38**, 161–176 (1961)

Bhagwat, A.G., Wong, P.: Effect of pH in direct OsO_4 fixation on glycogen staining as shown by electron microscopy; Stain Technol. **47**, 39–40 (1972)

Bignami, A., Dahl, D.: Astrocyte-specific protein and neuroglial response to injury in the cerebral cortex of the rat. Boston: 50th Annual Meeting of the American Association of Neuropathologists, 1974

Blakemore, W.F.: The fate of escaped plasma protein after thermol necrosis of the rat brain: an electron microscope study. J. Neuropathol. exp. Neurol. **28**, 139–152 (1969)

Bo, W.J., Smith, M.S.: A histochemical and biochemical study of phosphorylase and glycogen synthetase in smooth muscle, Anat. Rec. **153**, 295–302 (1965)

Bodian, D.: An electron-microscopic study of the monkey spinal cord, Bull. Johns Hopkins Hosp. **114**, 13–119 (1964)

Breckenridge, B.M., Crawford, E.J.: The quantitative histochemistry of the brain. Enzymes of glycogen metabolism, J. Neurochem. **7**, 234–240 (1961)

Breckenridge, B.M., Johnston, R.E.: Cyclic-3′,5′-nucleotide phosphodiesterase in brain, J. Histochem. Cytochem. **17**, 505–511 (1969)

Breckenridge, B.M., Norman, J.H.: Glycogen phosphorylase in brain. J. Neurochem. **9**, 383–392 (1962)

Breckenridge, B.M., Norman, J.H.: The conversion of phosphorylase b to phosphorylase a in brain, J. Neurochem., **12**, 51–57 (1965)

Bresciani, F., Auricchio, F., Fiore, C.: Effect of X-rays on movements of sodium in human erythrocytes. Radiat. Res. **21**, 394–412 (1964)

Broniszewska-Ardlet, B., Jongkind, J.F.: Effect of hypoxia on substrate levels in the brain of the adult mouse, J. Neurochem. **18**, 2237–2240 (1971)

Brown, A.W., Brierley, J.B.: The nature, distribution and earliest stages of anoxic-ischaemic nerve cell damage in the rat brain as defined by the optical microscope, Brit. J. exp. Pathol. **49**, 87–106 (1968)

Brown, A.W., Brierley, J.B.: Anoxic-ischaemic cell change in rat brain. Light microscopic and fine-structural observations. J. neurol. Sci. **16**, 59–84 (1972)

Bruijn, W.C. de: Glycogen, its chemistry and morphologic appearance in the electron micros-cope. I.A. modified OsO_4 fixative which selectively contrasts glycogen. J. Ultrastruct. Res. **42**, 29–50 (1973)

Brunner, E.A., Passonneau, J., Molstad, C.: The effect of volatile anaesthetics on levels of metabolites and on metabolic rate in brain. J. Neurochem. **18**, 2301–2316 (1971)

Bulmer, D.: Dimedone as an aldehyde blocking reagent to facilitate the histochemical de-monstration of glycogen. Stain Technol. **34**, 95–98 (1959)

Burns, J., Neame, P. B.: Staining of blood cells with periodic acid/salicyloyl hydrazide (PAS-SH). A fluorescent method for demonstrating glycogen. Blood 28, 674–682 (1966)

Calvo, W., Forteza-Vila, J.: Glycogen changes in bone marrow nerves after whole-body X-irradiation. Acta neuropathol. (Berl.) 20, 78–83 (1972)

Carter, S. H., Stone, W. E.: Effect of convulsants on brain glycogen in the mouse. J. Neurochem. 7, 16–19 (1961)

Chase, R. R.: Structural changes in the external geniculate body of rat following removal of eyes. Arch. Ophthalmol. 30, 75–86 (1943)

Chesler, A., Himwich, H. E.: The glycogen content of various parts of the central nervous system of dogs and cats at different ages. Arch. Biochem. Biophys. 2, 175–181 (1943)

Cheung, W. Y.: Cyclic nucleotide phosphodiesterase. p. 51–65. In: P. Greengard, E. Costa (Eds.). Advances in Biochemical Psychopharmacology. Vol. 3. New York: Raven Press. 1970

Chiang, J., Kowada, M., Ames, III, A., Wright, R. L., Majno, G.: Cerebral ischaemia, Part 3 (Vascular changes), Amer. J. Pathol. 52, 455–476 (1968)

Childress, C. C., Sacktor, B., Grossman, I. W., Bueding, E.: Isolation, ultrastructure, and biochemical characterization of glycogen in insect flight muscle. J. Cell Biol. 45, 83–90 (1970)

Cobb, J. D.: Calcification of rat cartilage and bone. Anat. Rec. 103, 531–532 (1949)

Cobb, J. D., Lafayette, W.: Relation of glycogen, phosphorylase and ground substance to calcifiction of bone. Arch. Path. 55, 496–505 (1953)

Cori, G. T., Cori, C. F.: Crystalline muscle phosphorylase IV. Formation of glycogen. J. biol. Chem. 151, 57–63 (1943)

Crowell, R. M., Olsson, Y.: Impaired microvascular filling after focal cerebral ischaemia in monkeys. J. Neurosurg. 36, 303–309 (1972)

Crowell, R. M., Olsson, Y., Klatzo, I., Ommaya, A. K.: Temporary occlusion of the middle cerebral artery in the monkey: clinical and pathological observations. Stroke 1, 439–448 (1970)

Crowell, R. M., Olsson, Y., Ommaya, A. K.: Angiographic and micrographic observations in experimental cerebral infarction. Neurology (Minneap.) 21, 710–719 (1971)

Cznarecki, C. M.: The effect of fixation on the chemical extraction of glycogen from rat liver. Histochem. J. 3, 163–167 (1971)

Daw, J. C., Berne, R. M.: Effect of sympathectomy on cardiac UDP-glycogen transferase activity in the cat. Amer. J. Physiol. 213, 1480–1484 (1967)

Dawes, G. S.: Comments about brain circulation, oxygen supply and anoxic survival. In: J. P. Schadé and W. H. McMenemey (Eds.), p. 37–40. Selective Vulnerability of The Brain In Hypoxaemia, F. A. Davis Co., Philadelphia, (1963)

Detrick, L. E.: Mucopolysaccharides in post-irradiation intestinal absorption studies. Ann. N.Y. Acad. Sci. 106, 636–645 (1963)

Drochmans, P., Dantan, E.: Size distributions of liver glycogen particles. p. 187–201. In: W. J. Wheland (Ed.), Control of Glycogen Metabolism. London-New York: Academic Press 1968

Drummond, G. I., Bellward, G.: Studies on phosphorylase b kinase from neural tissues. J. Neurochem. 17, 475–482 (1970)

Duffy, T. E., Nelson, S. R., Lowry, O. H.: Cerebral carbohydrate metabolism during acute hypoxia and recovery. J. Neurochem. 19, 959–977 (1972)

Dunkerley, G. B., Duncan, D.: A light and electron microscopic study of the normal and the degenerating corticospinal tract in the rat. J. comp. Neurol. 137, 155–184 (1969)

Eager, R. P., Eager, P. R.: Glial responses to degenerating cerebellar cortico-nuclear pathways in the cat. Science 153, 553–555 (1966)

Eckner, F. A. O.: Demonstration of phosphorylase and uridine diphosphate glucose-glycosyl transferase activities. J. Histochem. Cytochem. 19, 133 (1971)

Eckner, F. A. O., Riebe, B. H., Moulder, P. V., Blackstone, E. H.: Histochemical study of enzyme systems in frozen dried tissue. Histochemie 13, 283–288 (1968)

Eckner, F. A. O., Riebe, B. H., Moulder, P. V., Blackstone, E. H.: Polysaccharide synthesis in tissue sections. Evaluation of methods as an example of quality control in histochemistry. Histochemie 19, 340–354 (1969)

Edwards, C., Nahorski, S. R., Rogers, K. J.: In vivo changes of cerebral cyclic adenosine 3′,5′-monophosphate induced by biogenic amines: association with phosphorylase activation. J. Neurochem. 22, 565–572 (1974)

Edwards, C., Rogers, K.J.: Some factors influencing brain glycogen in the neonate chick. J. Neurochem. **19**, 2759–2766 (1972)

Egaña, E.: Aerobic and anaerobic metabolic studies of CNS exposed to internal radiation (P^{32}), p. 267. In: International Atomic Energy Agency. Effects of Ionizing Radiation on the Nervous System. Vienna: Christopher Resser's Söhne 1962

Eletskü, Yu.K.: Alteration of glycogen content in the brain of rats in acute alcoholic intoxication, Zh. Neuropatol. Psikhiatr. Im. S. S. Korsakova (in Russian) **63**, 1867–1873 (1963)

Eränkö, O., Palkama, A.: Improved localisation of phosphorylase by the use of polyvinyl pyrrolidone and high substrate concentration. J. Histochem. Cytochem. **9**, 585 (1961)

Estler, C.-J.: Der Glykogengehalt des Gehirns weißer Mäuse unter der Einwirkung von Phenobarbital und seine Beziehungen zu Blutzucker und Körpertemperatur. Med. exp. (Basel) **4**, 30–36 (1961a)

Estler, C.-J.: Glykogengehalt des Gehirns und Körpertemperatur weißer Mäuse unter dem Einfluß einziger zentral dämpfender und erregender Pharmaka. Med. exp. (Basel) **4**, 209–213 (1961b)

Estler, C.-J., Ammon, H.P.T.: The influence of the β-sympatheticolytic agent propranolol on glycogenolysis and glycolysis in muscle, brain and liver of white mice. Biochem. Pharmacol. **15**, 2031–2035 (1966)

Estler, C.-J., Ammon, H.P.T.: The influence of propranolol on the metamphetamine-induced changes of cerebral function and metabolism. J. Neurochem. **14**, 799–805 (1967)

Estler, C.-J., Heim, F.: Der Gehalt des Gehirns weißer Mäuse an Adeninnucleotiden, Kreatinphosphat, Coenzym A, Glykogen und Milchsäure in Ätherexcitation und -Narkose. Med. exp. (Basel). **3**, 241–248 (1960)

Fagundes, L.A., Cohen, R.B.: The effect of nutritional state on phosphorylase activity in the liver: A histochemical study. J. Histochem. Cytochem. **13**, 553–558 (1965)

Farkas-Bargeton, E., Olsson, Y., Guth, L., Klatzo, I.: Glycogen reaction to cerebral stab wound during maturation of rat brain. Acta neuropathol. (Berl.) **22**, 158–169 (1972)

Ferraro, A.: Experimental toxic encephalomyelopathy. Diffuse sclerosis following subcutaneous injections of potassium cyanide. Psychiat. Q. **7**, 267–283 (1933)

Filipova, V.N., Seits, I.F.: Effect of X-irradiation on the coenzyme A content of the bone marrow of rats, Dokl. Akad. Nauk. SSSR-Biol. Sci. Sect. (transl.), **154**, 1210–1213 (1964)

Fischer, E.H., Appleman, M.M., Krebs, E.G.: The structure of phosphorylases. p. 94–103. In: W.J. Whelan and M.P. Cameron (Eds.), Control of Glycogen Metabolism. London: J. & A. Churchill Ltd. 1964

Fischer, E.H., Hurd, S.S., Koh, P., Seery, V.L., Teller, D.C.: Phosphorylase: Relation of structure to activity p. 19–33. In: W.J. Whelan (Ed.), Control of Glycogen Metabolism, London, N.Y: Academic Press, 1968

Folbergrová, J.: Glycogen and glycogen phosphorylase in the cerebral cortex of mice under the influence of methionine sulphoximine. J. Neurochem. **20**, 547–557 (1973)

Folbergrová, J., Lowry, O.H., Passonneau, J.V.: Changes in metabolites of the energy reserves in individual layers of mouse cerebral cortex and subjacent white matter during ischaemia and anaesthesia. J. Neurochem. **17**, 1155–1162 (1970)

Folbergrová, J., Passonneau, J.V., Lowry, O.H., Schulz, D.W.: Glycogen, ammonia and related metabolites in the brain during seizures evoked by methionine sulphoximine. J. Neurochem. **16**, 191–203 (1969)

Fontaine, G., Résibois, A., Tondeur, M., Jonniaux, G., Farriaux, J.P., Voet, W., Maillard, E., Loeb, H.: Gangliosidosis with total hexosaminidase deficiency: clinical, biochemical and ultrastructural studies and comparison with conventional cases of Tay-Sachs disease. Acta neuropathol. (Berl.) **23**, 118–132 (1973)

Frank, G.M., Snezhko, A.D.: The rythm of oxidative processes and its disturbance under the action of radiation. p. 269–284. In: R.J.C. Harris (Ed.), The Initial Effects of Ionizing Radiations on Cells. London: Academic Press 1961

Franke, H., Lierse, H.: Elektronenmikroskopische Untersuchungen über Hirnveränderungen des Meerschweinchens nach Röntgenbestrahlung. Forsch. Röntgenstrahlen. **102**, 78–87 (1966)

French, D.: Structure of glycogen and its amylolytic degradation, p. 7–24. In: W.J. Whelan and M.P. Cameron (Eds.), Control of Glycogen Metabolism. London: Churchill 1964

Friede, R.L.: Über die trophische Funktion der Glia, Virchow's Arch. path. Anat. **324**, 15–26 (1953)

Friede, R.L.: Die Bedeutung der Glia für den zentralen Kohlenhydratstoffwechsel, Zentralbl. allg. Pathol. pathol. Anat. **92**, 65–74 (1954)

Friede, R.L.: Über Beziehungen zwischen histochemischen Glykogenbefunden und Hirn-wellenfrequenz im EEG an einem Material von menschlichen Biopsien, Arch. Psychiatr. Nervenkr., **194**, 213–237 (1956)

Friede, R.L.: Histochemical demonstration of phosphorylase in brain tissue: association of postmortal neuron changes with phosphorylase activity. J. Histochem. Cytochem, **7**, 34–38 (1959a)

Friede, R.L.: Histochemical distribution of phosphorylase in the brain of the guinea pig. J. Neurol. Neurosurg. Psychiatr. **22**, 325–329 (1959b)

Friede, R.L.: Correlations between the electroencephalogram and cortical histochemical changes in experimental brain lesions. Exp. Neurol. **5**, 89–99 (1962)

Friede, R.L.: Topographic Brain Chemistry. p. 132–157, New York: Academic Press 1966

Friede, R.L., Houten, W.H. van: Relations between postmortem alterations and glycolytic metabolism in the brain. Exp. Neurol. **4**, 197–204 (1961)

Fuentes, C., Marty, R.: Oligodendrocytose réactionelle au cours de la dégénérescence ex-périmentale du cortex cérébral. J. neurol. Sci. **10**, 535–540 (1970)

Gambetti, P., Mauro, S.Di., Baker, L.: Nervous system in Pompe's disease. Ultrastructure and biochemistry. J. Neuropathol. exp. Neurol. **30**, 412–430 (1971)

Gatfield, P.D., Lowry, O.H., Schulz, D.W., Passonneau, J.V.: Regional energy reserves in mouse brain and changes with ischaemia and anaesthesia. *J. Neurochem.* **13**, 185–195 (1966)

Gercken, G., Preuss, H.: The effect of breathing oxygen on the metabolism of the rat brain under normal and ischaemic conditions. *J. Neurochem.* **16**, 761–767 (1969)

Gerstner, H.B., Brooks, P.M., Vogel, F.S., Smith, S.A.: Effect of head X-irradiation in rabbits on aortic blood pressure, brain water content and cerebral histology. Radiat. Res. **5**, 318–331 (1956)

Gerstner, H.B., Kent, S.P.: Early effects of head X-irradiation in rabbits. Radiat. Res. **6**, 626–644 (1957)

Ginsburg, J.M., Ulmer, D.D.: Massive dose irradiation of the mammalian central nervous system. U.S. AMRL Report No. 339, 1958

Glees, P., Hasan, M., Tischner, K.: Ultrastructural features of transneuronal atrophy in monkey geniculate neurons. Acta neuropathol. (Berl.), **7**, 361–366 (1967)

Go, G., Berson, F., Klatzo, I., Spatz, M.: The effect of ischaemia and hypoxia on glucose transport in the brain. J. Neuropathol. exp. Neurol. **33**, 183–184 (1974)

Godlewski, H.G.: Are active and inactive phosphorylases histochemically distinguishable. J. Histochem. Cytochem. **11**, 108–112 (1963)

Goldberg, B., Wade, O.R., Jones, H.W., Jr.: Polysaccharide synthesis in frozen tissue sec-tions as a histochemical method for phosphorylase, J. nat. Cancer Inst., **13**, 543–557 (1952)

Goldberg, N.D., Lust, W.D., O'Dea, R.F., Wei, S., O'Toole, A.G.: A role of cyclic nucleotides in brain metabolism. Vol. 3, p. 67–87. In: P. Greengard and E. Costa (Eds.). Role of Cyclic AMP in Cell Function, Advances in Biochemical Psychopharmacology, New York: Raven Press 1970

Goldberg, N.D., O'Toole, A.G.: The properties of glycogen synthetase and regulation of glycogen biosynthesis in rat brain. J. biol. Chem. **244**, 3053–3061 (1969)

Grillo, T.A.I.: A histochemical study of phosphorylase in the tissues of the chick embryo. J. Histochem. Cytochem. **9**, 386–391 (1961)

Guha, S., Wegmann, R.: Phosphorylase in chick-embryo liver. J. Histochem. Cytochem. **9**, 454–455 (1961)

Guha, S., Wegmann, R.: Histoautoradiographic localization of phosphorylase activity. J. Histochem. Cytochem. **13**, 148–150 (1965)

Guha, S., Wegmann, R.: The use of C^{14}-labelled substrate in histochemical demonstration of different forms of phosphorylase. Histochemie, **6**, 350–361 (1966)

Guth, L., Watson, P.K.: A correlated histochemical and quantitative study on cerebral glycogen after brain injury in the rat. Exp. Neurol. **22**, 590–602 (1968)

Hager, H.: Die frühen Alterationen des Nervengewebes nach Hypoxidose und die fortge-schrittene Nekrose im elektronenmikroskopischen Bild. p. 64. In: F. Lüthy and A. Bi-schoff (Eds.). Proc. V Intern. Congr. Neuropath. Amsterdam: Excerpta Med. Found. 1966

Hager, H., Luh, S., Ruščáková, D., Rušcák, M.: Histochemische, elektronenmikroskopische und biochemische Untersuchungen über Glykogenhäufung in reaktiv veränderten Astro-zyten der traumatisch lädierten Säugergroßhirnrinde, Z. Zellforsch. **83**, 295–320 (1967)

Hamberger, A., Sjöstrand, J.: Respiratory enzyme activities in neurons and glial cells of the hypoglossal nucleus during nerve regeneration, Acta physiol. scand. 67, 76–88 (1966)

Hassid, W. Z., Doudoroff, M., Barker, H. A.: Phosphorylases-phosphorolysis and synthesis of saccharides. p. 1014. In: F. B. Sumner and K. Myrbäck (Eds.), The Enzymes (Part 2). New York: Academic Press 1951

Haymaker, W.: Effects of ionizing radiation on nervous tissue, p. 441–518. In: G. H. Bourne (Ed.), The Structure and Function of Nervous Tissue, Vol. III, New York: Academic Press 1970

Haymaker, W., Ibrahim, M. Z. M., Miquel, J., Call, N., Noden, P., Ashley, W., Ballinger, E. R., Ghidoni, J., Lindsay, I. R., Behar, A. J., Baker, G.: Acute changes in the central nervous system of monkeys exposed to protons, J. Neuropathol. exp. Neurol. 31, 72–101 (1972)

Haymaker, W., Miquel, J., Ibrahim, M. Z. M.: Glycogen accumulation following brain trauma. p. 71–87. In: H. T. Wycis (Ed.), Current Research in Neurosciences, Basel, New York: Karger 1970

Helmreich, E., Michaelidis, M. C., Cori, C. F.: Effects of substrates and a substrate analog on the binding of 5'-adenylic acid to muscle phosphorylase. Biochemistry (Wash.) 6, 3695–3710 (1967)

Henion, W. F., Sutherland, E. W.: Immunological differences of phosphorylases J. biol. Chem. 224, 477–488 (1957)

Hers, H. G., Wulf, H. de: The regulation of glycogen synthesis in the liver, p. 65–76. In: W. J. Whelan (Ed.), Control of Glycogen Metabolism New York: Academic Press 1968

Hess, A.: Blood-brain barrier and ground substance of central nervous system. Arch. Neurol. Psychiatr. 74, 149–157 (1955)

Hess, R., Pearse, A. G. E.: Dissociation of uridine diphosphate glucose-glycogen transglucosylase from phosphorylase activity in individual muscle fibers. Proc. Soc. exp. Biol. Med. 107, 569–571 (1961)

Hicks, S. P.: Brain metabolism in vivo. (I) The distribution of lesions caused by cyanide poisoning, insulin hypoglycaemia, asphyxia in nitrogen and fluroacetate poisoning in rats. Arch. Pathol. (Chicago), 49, 111–137 (1950)

Hills, C. P.: Ultrastructural changes in the capillary bed of the rat cerebral cortex in anoxic-ischaemic brain lesions. Amer. J. Pathol. 44, 531–552 (1964)

Hirano, A., Levine, S., Zimmerman, H.: Experimental cyanide encephalopathy: electron microscopic observations of early lesions in white matter. J. Neuropathol. exp. Neurol. 26, 200–213 (1967)

Hoffmann, P. C., Toon, R., Kleinman, J., Heller, A.: The association of lesion-induced reductions in brain monoamines with alterations in striatal carbohydrate metabolism. J. Neurochem. 20, 69–80 (1973)

Hori, S. H.: Cytological phosphorylase locations in rat liver and muscle as shown by a lead precipitation method, Stain Technol. 39, 275–278 (1964)

Hori, S. H.: Effect of EDTA on histochemical demonstration of phosphorylase activity. J. Histochem. Cytochem. 14, 501–508 (1966a)

Hori, S. H.: Fine-structure locations of α-glucan phosphorylase, as shown by lead precipitation and electron microscopy. Stain Technol. 41, 91–95 (1966b)

Hornbrook, K. R., Brody, T. M.: The effect of catecholamines on muscle glycogen and phosphorylase activity. J. Pharmacol. exp. Ther. 140, 295–307 (1963)

Houten, W. H. van, Friede, R. L.: Histochemical studies of cyanide demyelination produced with cyanide. Exp. Neurol. 4, 402–412 (1961)

Huang, M., Shimizu, H., Daly, J.: Regulation of adenosine cyclic-3',5'-phosphate formation in cerebral cortical slices. Interaction among norepinephrine, histamine, serotonin. Molec. Pharmacol. 7, 155–162 (1971)

Hultborn, R., Jarlstedt, J.: Effect of ethanol on the oxygen consumption of cerebral cortex, cerebellar cortex and liver homogenates. J. Neuropathol. exp. Neurol. 33, 107–112 (1974)

Hurst, E. W.: A review of some recent observations on demyelination. Brain 67, 103–124 (1944)

Husain, S., Paradise, R. R.: Effect of halothane on CO_2 production from glucose, frctose and pyruvate in rat cerebral cortical slices. J. Neurochem. 21, 1161–1166 (1973)

Hutchins, D., Rogers, K. J.: Physiological and drug-induced changes in the glycogen content of mouse brain. Brit. J. Pharmacol. Chemother. 39, 9–25 (1970)

Hutchinson, B. T., Kuwabara, T.: Phosphorylase and uridine diphosphoglucose glycogen synthetase in the retina. Arch. Ophthalmol. 68, 538–545 (1962)

Hydén, H.: The nueron and its glia—a biochemical and functional unit. Endeavour **21**, 144–155 (1962)

Hydén, H.: Dynamic aspects of the neuron-glia relationship—a study with microchemical methods, p. 179–219. In: H. Hydén (Ed.), The Neuron Amsterdam: Elsevier Publ. Co. 1967

Ibrahim, M. Z. M.: Postmortem changes in active and total phosphorylase of the rat brain, p. 113–115. In: 3rd International Congress of Histochemistry and Cytochemistry, Berlin-Heidelberg-New York: Springer 1968

Ibrahim, M. Z. M.: The response of the brain to hypoxia and ischaemia. J. neurol. Sci. **17**, 271–279 (1972)

Ibrahim, M. Z. M.: The mast cells of the mammalian central nervous system, Part 2 (The effect of proton irradiation in the monkey). J. neurol. Sci. **21**, 479–499 (1974)

Ibrahim, M. Z. M., Atlan, H., Miquel, J., Castellani, P., Synthetic and hydrolytic enzymes of glycogen in the normal and the irradiated rat brain. Radiat. Res. **43**, 341–355 (1970a)

Ibrahim, M. Z. M., Briscoe, P. B. Jr., Bayliss, O. B., Adams, C. W. M.: The relationship between enzyme activity and neuroglia in the prodromal and demyelinating stages of cyanide encephalopathy in the rat. J. Neurol. Neurosurg. Psychiatr. **26**, 479–486 (1963)

Ibrahim, M. Z. M., Castellani, P.: Demonstration of phosphorylase activity in the rat brain. Histochemie **16**, 9–14 (1968)

Ibrahim, M. Z. M., Khreis, Y., Koshayan, D. S.: The histochemical identification of microglia. J. neurol. Sci. **22**, 211–233 (1974)

Ibrahim, M. Z. M., Levine, S.: The effect of cyanide intoxication on the metachromatic material found in the central nervous system. J. Neurol. Neurosurg. Psychiatr. **30**, 545–555 (1967)

Ibrahim, M. Z. M., Miquel, J., Haymaker, W.: Glycogen, phosphorylase and branching enzyme in experimental and pathological conditions of the rat brain. J. Neuropathol. exp. Neurol. **27**, 119 (1968)

Ibrahim, M. Z. M., Pascoe, E., Alam, S., Miquel, J.: Glycogen and phosphorylase activity in rat brain during recovery from several forms of hypoxia. Amer. J. Pathol. **60**, 403–420 (1970b)

Ibrahim, M. Z. M., Pascoe, E., Khayat, M. Y. N.: Histochemical evidence for phosphorylase, branching enzyme and glycogen synthetase activities in rat brain. J. neurol. Sci. **19**, 117–131 (1973)

Ito, U., Go, G., Spatz, M., Klatzo, I.: Cerebrovascular reactions to ischemia in the mongolian gerbil. J. Neuropathol. exp. Neurol. **33**, 184 (1974)

Jirmanová, I.: Glycogen deposits in motorneurons of young chickens following peripheral nerve section. Acta neuropathol. (Berl.) **19**, 110–120 (1971)

Joseph, J.: Nuclear population changes in degenerating posterior columns of rabbit's spinal cord. Acta anat. (Basel) **21**, 356–365 (1954)

Kahn, V., Blum, J. J.: The glycogen phosphorylase of Tetrahymena pyriformis. II. Inhibition and inactivation by EDTA and ATP and other kinetic properties. Arch. Biochem. Biophys, **143**, 92–105 (1971)

Kakiuchi, S., Rall, T. W.: The influence of chemical agents on the accumulation of adenosine-3′,5′-phosphate in slices of rabbit cerebellum. Molec. Pharmacol. **4**, 367–378 (1968a)

Kakiuchi, S., Rall, T. W.: Studies of adenosine-3′,5′-phosphate in rabbit cerebral cortex. Molec. Pharmacol. **4**, 379–388 (1968b)

Karlsberg, P., Adams, J. E., Elliot, H. W.: Inhibition and reversal of serotonin-induced cerebral vasospasm. Surg. Forum. **13**, 425–427 (1962)

Kay, R. E., Chan, H.: Effect of X-irradiation on glucose metabolism in rat cerebral cortex slices. J. Neurochem. **14**, 401–403 (1967)

Kay, R. E., Entenman, C.: Hyperglycaemia and increased liver glycogen in rats after X-irradiation. Proc. Soc. exp. Biol. Med. (N.Y.) **91**, 143–146 (1956)

Kerr, S. E., Antaki, A.: The carbohydrate metabolism of brain. (V) The effect of certain narcotics and convulsant drugs upon the carbohydrate and phosphocreatine content of rabbit brain. J. biol. Chem. **122**, 49–52 (1937)

Kerr, S. E., Ghantus, M.: The carbohydrate metabolism of brain (II) The effect of varying the carbohydrate and insulin supply on the glycogen, free sugar and lactic acid in the mammalian brain. J. biol. Chem. **116**, 9–20 (1936)

Kety, S. S.: Regional circulation of the brain under physiological conditions—possible relationship to selective vulnerability. p. 21–26. In: J. P. Schadé and W. H. McMenemey (Eds.), Selective Vulnerability of the Brain in Hypoxaemia, Philadelphia: Davis 1963

Khan, T., Green, B., Raimondi, A.J.: Energy metabolism of acutely injured spinal cord of cat. 50th Annual Meeting of the American Association of Neuropathologists, Boston. 1974

King, L.J., Carl, J.L., Lao, L.: Carbohydrate metabolism in brain during convulsions and its modification by phenobarbitone. J. Neurochem. **20**, 477–485 (1973)

Klatzo, I., Farkas-Bargeton, E., Guth, L., Miquel, J., Olsson, Y.: Some morphological and biochemical aspects of abnormal glycogen accumulation in the glia, p. 351–365. In: Proc. 6th International Congress of Neuropathology (Paris), Paris: Masson & Cie 1970

Klatzo, I., Miquel, J., Tobias, C., Haymaker, W.: Effects of alpha particle radiation on the rat brain, including vascular permeability and glycogen studies. J. Neuropathol. exp. Neurol. **20**, 459–483 (1961)

Koizumi, J., Shiraishi, H.: Ultrastructural appearance of glycogen in the hypothalamus of the rabbit following chlorpromazine administration. Exp. Brain Res. **10**, 276–282 (1970)

Korsgaard, B., Wulff, H.R.: An improved method for the histochemical demonstration of phosphorylase in tissue sections. Acta pathol. microbiol. scand. **70**, 236–240 (1967)

Köver, G., Schoffeniels, E.: Effets de l'irradiation X et de différentes substances sur les caractères de perméabilité des hématies. Internat. J. Radiat. Biol. **9**, 461–476 (1966)

Krebs, E.G., Fischer, E.H.: Molecular properties and transformations of glycogen phosphorylase in animal tissues. Adv. Enzym. **24**, 263–290 (1962)

Krebs, E.G., Fischer, E.H.: Phosphorylase and related enzymes of glycogen metabolism. Vitam. Horm. **22**, 399–410 (1964)

Krebs, E.G., Love, D.S., Bratvold, G.E., Trayser, K.A., Meyer, W.L., Fischer, E.H.: Purification and properties of rabbit skeletal muscle phosphorylase b kinase. Biochemistry (Wash.), **3**, 1022–1033 (1964)

Krug, A., Dharamadhach, A., Krug, Ch.: Zum histochemischen Phosphorylasenachweis im Herzinfarct. Histochemie **10**, 376–377 (1967)

Kumamoto, T.: Histochemical studies in the changes of brain glycogen caused by starvation, Osaka Daigaku Igaku Zasski, **5**, 553–562 (in Japanese), Cited by R.L. Friede (1966) Topographic Brain Chemistry. p. 142. New York: Academic Press 1953

Kuwabara, T., Cogan, D.G.: Retinal glycogen. Arch. Ophthalmol. **66**, 680–688 (1961)

Lampert, P.W.: A comparative electron microscopic study of reactive degenerating, regenerating and dystrophic axons. J. Neuropathol. exp. Neurol. **26**, 345–368 (1967)

Lampert, P.W., Fox, J.L., Earle, K.M.: Cerebral edema after laser radiation. An electron microscopic study, J. Neuropathol. exp. Neurol. **25**, 531–541 (1966)

Lampert, P.W., O'Brien, J., Garrett, R.: Hexachlorophene encephalopathy. Acta neuropathol. (Berl.) **23**, 326–333 (1973)

Larner, J., Villar-Palasi, C., Goldberg, N.D., Bishop, J.S., Huijing, F., Wenger, J.I., Sasko, H., Brown, N.B.: Hormonal and nonhormonal control of glycogen synthesis-control of transferase phosphatase and transferase I kinase, p. 1–18. In: W.J. Whelan (Ed.), Control of Glycogen Metabolism, New York: Academic Press, 1968

Lazarow, A.: Particulate glycogen: A submicroscopic component of the guinea pig liver cell; its significance in glycogen storage and the regulation of blood sugar. Anat. Rec. **84**, 31–50 (1942)

Le Fevre, P.G., Peters, A.A.: Evidence of mediated transfer of monosaccharides from blood to brain in rodents. J. Neurochem. **13**, 35–46 (1966)

Leloir, L.F.: Rôle of uridine diphosphate glucose in the synthesis of glycogen, p. 68–81. In: W.J. Whelan and M.P. Cameron (Eds.), Control of Glycogen Metabolism. London: Churchill 1964

Leske, R., Mayersbach, H.V.: The role of histochemical and biochemical preparation methods for the detection of glycogen. J. Histochem. Cytochem. **17**, 527–538 (1969)

Levine, S.: Anoxic-ischaemic encephalopathy in rats. Amer. J. Pathol. **36**, 1–17 (1960)

Levine, S., Klein, M.: Ischaemic infarction and swelling in the rat brain. Arch. Pathol. **69**, 544–553 (1960)

Levine, S., Stypulkowski, W.: Experimental cyanide encephalopathy. Arch. Pathol. **67**, 306–323 (1959)

Lindberg, L.-A., Palkama, A.: Methodological observations on the histochemical demonstration of glycogen phosphorylase activity. Ann. Med. exp. Biol. Fenn. **48**, 67–76 (1970a)

Lindberg, L.-A., Palkama, A.: Histochemical demonstration of phosphorylase with lead technique; real or artifact. Scand. J. clin. Lab. Invest. **25**, suppl. 113, p. 75 (1970b)

Lindberg, L.-A., Palkama, A.: The effect of some factors on the histochemical demonstration of liver glycogen phosphorylase activity, J. Histochem. Cytochem. **20**, 331–335 (1972)

Lindberg, R.: Patterns of CNS vulnerability in acute hypoxaemia, including anaesthesia accidents, p. 189–209. In: J.P. Schadé and W.H. McMenemey (Eds.), Selective Vulnerability of the Brain in Hypoxaemia, Philadelphia: Davis 1969

Long, D.M., Maxwell, R.E., French, L.A.: The effects of glucosteroids upon cold-induced brain edema. III. Prevertion of gliosis following brain edema. J. Neuropathol. exp. Neurol. 32, 245–255 (1973)

Long, D.M., Mossakowski, M.J., Klatzo, I.: Glycogen accumulation in spinal motor neurons due to partial ischemia, Acta neuropathol. (Berl.) 20, 335–347 (1972)

Loutit, J.F.: Biological action of radiation, Lectures on the Scientific Basis of Medicine 1, 379–396 (1952)

Lowry, O., Passonneau, J.V., Hasselberger, F.X., Schulz, D.W.: Effect of ischaemia on known substrates and cofactors of the glycolytic pathway in brain, J. biol. Chem. 239, 18–31 (1964)

Lucas, B.G.B., Strangeways, D.H.: Experimental cerebral anoxia, J. Pathol. Bact. 86, 273–281 (1963)

Lumsden, C.E.: Cyanide leucoencephalopathy in rats and observations on the vascular and ferment hypotheses of demyelinating diseases. J. Neurol. Neurosurg. Psychiatr. 13, 1–15 (1950)

Lundgren, P.R., Miquel, J.: The incorporation of isotopic carbon C^{14} into the cerebral glycogen of normal and X-irradiated rats. J. Neurochem. 17, 1383–1386 (1970)

Maas, H., Schubert, G.: Early biochemical reactions after X-irradiation, Vol. 22, p. 449–454. In: Proceedings of the Second U.N. International Conference on the Peaceful Uses of Atomic Energy, Geneva: United Nations 1958

MacMillan, V., Siesjö, B.K.: The effect of phenobarbitone anaesthesia upon some organic phosphates, glycolytic metabolites and citric acid cycle-associated intermediates of the rat brain. J. Neurochem. 20, 1669–1681 (1973)

Maker, H.S., Lehrer, G.M., Weiss, C., Silides, D.J., Scheinberg, L.C.: The quantitative histochemistry of a chemically induced ependymoblastoma. Part 2 (The effect of ischaemia on substrates of carbohydrate metabolism). J. Neurochem. 13, 1207–1212 (1966)

Manners, D.J.: Branching enzymes. p. 83–100. In: W.J. Whelan (Ed.), Control of Glycogen Metabolism. New York: Academic Press 1968

Marinesco, G.: Sur la presence et les variations du glycogéne dans le névraxe et les glandes endocrines (A l'état normal et pathologique). Ann. Anat. Path. Medicochirurgicale, 5, 233–250 (1928). Cited by R.L. Friede, Topographic Brain Chemistry, p. 141. New York: Academic Press 1966

Martin, D.L., Engel, W.K.: Dependency of histochemical phosphorylase staining on amount of cellular glycogen. J. Histochem. Cytochem. 20, 476–479 (1972)

Martin, J.J., Barsy, Th. de, Hoof, F. Van, Palladini, G.: Pompe's disease: an inborn lysosomal disorder with storage of glycogen. Acta neuropathol. (Berl.) 23, 229–244 (1973)

Mayman, C.I., Gatfield, P.D., Breckenridge, B.M.: The glucose content of brain in anaesthesia. J. Neurochem. 11, 483–487 (1964)

MacDonald, M., Spector, R.G.: The influence of anoxia on respiratory enzymes in rat brain. Brit. J. exp. Pathol. 44, 11–15 (1963)

McGee-Russell, S.M., Brown, A.W., Brierley, J.B.: A combined light and electron microscope study of early anoxic-ischaemic cell change in rat brain. Brain Res. 20, 193–200 (1970)

Meijer, A.E.F.H.: Improved histochemical method for the demonstration of the activity of α-glucan phosphorylase. (I) The use of glucosyl acceptor. Histochemie 12, 244–252 (1968a)

Meijer, A.E.F.H.: Improved histochemical method for the demonstration of the activity of α-glucan phosphorylase. (II) Relation of molecular weight of glucosyl acceptor dextran to activation of phosphorylase. Histochemie 16, 134–143 (1968b)

Melching, H.-J.: The influence of serotonin on radiation effects in mammals. Vol. 1, p. 93–137. In: M. Ebert and A. Howard (Eds.), Current Topics in Radiation Research, Amsterdam: North Holland Publishing Co. 1965

Mellerup, E.T.: Brain glycogen after intracisternal injection of some corticosteroids. J. Neurochem. 17, 607–611 (1970)

Mellerup, E.T., Rafaelsen, O.J.: Brain glycogen after intracisternal insulin injection. J. Neurochem. 16, 777–781 (1969)

Meyer, A.: Intoxications, p. 235. In: W. Blackwood, W.H. McMenemey, A. Meyer, R.M. Norman and D.S. Russell (Eds.). Neuropathology. Baltimore, Md.: Wiliams and Wilkins 1963

Meyer, J. S.: Circulatory changes following occlusion of the middle cerebral artery and their relation to function. J. Neurosurg. **15**, 653–673 (1958)

Meyer, J. S., Portnoy, H. D.: Localized cerebral hypoglycemia simulating stroke. Neurology (Minneap.) **8**, 601–614 (1958)

Mihailović, L. T., Čupić, D., Dekleva, N.: Changes in the numbers of neurons and glial cells in the lateral geniculate nucleus of the monkey during retrograde cell degeneration. J. comp. Neurol. **142**, 223–229 (1971)

Miquel, J., Haymaker, W.: Astroglial reaction to ionizing radiation. Progr. Brain Res. **15**, 89–114 (1965)

Miquel, J., Haymaker, W.: Glycogen accumulation in monkey and cat brain exposed to proton radiation, p. 792–797. In: F. Luthy and A. Bischoff (Eds.). Proceedings of the Vth International Congress of Neuropathology, Excerpta Medica (Amst.), 1966

Miquel, J., Klatzo, I., Menzel, D. B., Haymaker, W.: Glycogen changes in X-irradiated rat brain. Acta neuropath. (Berl.) **2**, 482–490 (1963)

Mori, S., Leblond, C. P.: Electron microscopic features and proliferation of astrocytes in the corpus callosum of the rat. J. comp. Neurol. **137**, 197–226 (1969)

Mossakowski, M. J., Long, D. M., Myers, R. E., Curet, H. R. de, Klatzo, I.: Early histochemical and ultrastructural changes in perinatal asphyxia. J. Neuropathol. exp. Neurol. **27**, 500–516 (1968)

Mršulja, B. B.: Cyclic nucleotides and brain glycogen. Experientia (Basel) **30**, 66–68 (1974)

Mršulja, B. B., Rakic, Lj. M., Micic, D.: Possible form of glycogen bound in phosphatidopeptides in the brain. J. Neurochem. **15**, 1377–1379 (1968)

Nair, V.: Regional changes in brain serotonin after head X-irradiation and its significance in the potentiation of barbiturate hypnosis. Nature (Lond.), **208**, 1293–1294 (1965)

Narang, H. K., Field, E. J.: An electron-microscopic study of multiple sclerosis biopsy material: some unusual inclusions. J. neurol. Sci. **18**, 287–300 (1973)

Nelson, S. R., Schulz, D. W., Passonneau, J. V., Lowry, O. H.: Control of glycogen levels in brain. J. Neurochem. **15**, 1271–1279 (1968)

Niemeyer, H., Perez, N., Garces, E., Vergara, F. E.: Enzyme synthesis in mammalian liver as a consequence of refeeding after fasting. Biochim. Biophys. Acta **62**, 411–413 (1962)

Niemi, M.: The retina and its diseases, p. 599–621. In: C. W. M. Adams (Ed.), Neurohistochemistry, Elsevier 1965

Noak, W., Wolff, J. R., Güldner, F.-H., Moritz, A.: Über die akuten Veränderungen in Parietalcortex der Ratte nach spitzem Trauma. Acta neuropath. (Berl.) **19**, 249–264 (1971)

Oksche, A.: Der histochemisch nachweisbare Glykogenaufbau und -abbau in den Astrozyten und Ependymzellen als Beispiel einer funktionsabhängigen Stoffwechselaktivität der Neuroglia. Z. Zellforsch. **54**, 307–361 (1961)

Paasonen, M. K.: Release of 5-hydroxytryptamine from blood platelets. J. Pharm. Pharmacol. **17**, 681–697 (1965)

Paasonen, M. K., MacLean, P. D., Giarman, N. J.: 5-Hydroxytryptamine (serotonin, enteramine) content of structures of the limbic system. J. Neurochem. **1**, 326–333 (1957)

Palaić, D. J., Supek, Z.: Liberation of brain 5-hydroxytryptamine and noradrenaline by X-ray treatment in the newborn and adult rat. J. Neurochem. **13**, 705–709 (1966)

Palmer, G. C., Schmidt, M. J., Robison, G. A.: Development and characteristics of the histamine-induced accumulation of cyclic AMP in the rabbit cerebral cortex. J. Neurochem. **19**, 2251–2256 (1972)

Palmer, G. C., Sulser, F., Robison, G. A.: The effects of neurohumoral agents on the level of cyclic AMP in different brain areas *in vitro*. Pharmacologist **11**, 258 (1969)

Papa, S., Secchi, A. G., Lofrumento, N. E., D'Ermo, F., Quagliariello, E.: Oxidative phosphorylation in retina mitochondria. Ital. J. Biochem. (Engl. Ed.) **14**, 174–183 (1965)

Parmeggiani, A., Morgan, H. E.: Effect of adenine nucleotides and inorganic phosphate on muscle phosphorylase activity. Biochem. biophys. Res. Commun. **9**, 252–256 (1962)

Passonneau, J. V., Brunner, E. A., Molstad, C., Passonneau, R.: The effects of altered endocrine states and of ether anaesthesia on mouse brain. J. Neurochem. **18**, 2317–2328 (1971)

Passonneau, J. V., Lowry, O. H.: Phosphofructokinase and the Pasteur effect. Biochem. biophys. Res. Commun. **7**, 10–15 (1962)

Pearse, A. G. E.: Histochemistry, Theoretical and Applied. vol. 1, 3rd ed., Boston, N.Y.: Little, Brown and Co. 1968

Pearse, A. G. E.: Histochemistry Theoretical and Applied, vol. 2, 3rd ed., Boston, N.Y.: Little, Brown and Co. 1972

Piras, M.M. De, Zadunaisky, J.A.: Effect of potassium and ouabain on glucose metabolism by frog brain. J. Neurochem. **12**, 657–661 (1965)

Plum, F., Posner, J.B., Alvord, E.C. Jr: Edema and necrosis in experimental cerebral infarction. Arch. Neurol. (Chic.) **9**, 563–570 (1963)

Pontén, U., Ratcheson, R.A., Siesjö, B.K.: Metabolic changes in the brains of mice frozen in liquid nitrogen. J. Neurochem. **21**, 1121–1126 (1973)

Prasannan, K.G., Subrahmanyam, K.: Effect of insulin on the glycogen synthesis *in vivo* in the brain and liver of rats under different conditions. Indian J. med. Res. **53**, 1003–1009 (1965)

Prasannan, K.G., Subrahmanyam, K.: Effect of insulin on the synthesis of glycogen in cerebral cortical slices of alloxan diabetic rats. Endocrinology **82**, 1–6 (1968a)

Prasannan, K.G., Subrahmanyam, K.: Enzymes of glycogen metabolism in cerebral cortex of normal and diabetic rats. J. Neurochem. **15**, 1239–1241 (1968b)

Pronaszko-Kurczyńska, A., Mossakowski, M.J., Ostenda, M., Korthals, J.: Changes in brain glycogen content in experimental ischemia. Neuropatol. pol. **9**, 281–294 (1971)

Raine, C.S., Hummelgard, A., Swanson, E., Bornstein, M.B.: Multiple sclerosis: serum-induced demyelination *in vitro*. A light and electron microscope study. J. neurol. Sci. **20**, 127–148 (1973)

Rajan, R., Prasannan, K.G., Subrahmanyam, K.: Effect of cortisone on the levels of glycogen in the brain and liver of the fasting rat. Indian J. med. Res. **57**, 933–936 (1963)

Rall, T.W., Sattin, A.: Factors influencing the accumulation of cyclic AMP in brain tissue, Vol. 3, p. 113–133. In: P. Greengard and E. Costa (Eds.), Role of Cyclic AMP in Cell Function. Advances in Biochemical Psycho-pharmacology, New York: Raven Press 1970

Raynor, R.B., McMurtry, J.G., Pool, J.L.: Cerebrovascular effects of topically applied serotonin in the cat. Neurology (Minneap.) **11**, 190–195 (1961)

Renson, J., Fischer, P.: Libération de 5-hyroxytryptamine par le rayonnement X. Arch. int. Physiol. Biochem. **67**, 142–144 (1959)

Revel, J.P.: Electron microscopy of glycogen. J. Histochem. Cytochem. **12**, 104–114 (1964)

Ribadeau-Dumas, J.L., Escourolle, R., Castaigne, P.: Syndrome de Creutzfeldt-Jakob: Étude ultrastructurale de trois observations. Rev. neurol. (Paris) **121**, 405–422 (1969)

Rivera, A., Jr., Brann, A.W., Jr., Myers, R.E.: Brain glycogen of the recovering asphyxiated monkey newborn. Exp. Neurol. **26**, 309–315 (1970)

Roach, M.K., Reese, W.N., Jr.: Effect of ethanol on glucose and amino acid metabolism in brain. Biochem. Pharmacol. **20**, 2805–2812 (1971)

Robinson, N.: Histochemistry of enzyme response to trauma in the neocortex and corpus callosum of developing rat brain. J. Neurol. Neurosurg. Psychiatr. **36**, 1046–1052 (1973)

Robison, G.A., Schmidt, M.J., Sutherland, E.W.: On the development and properties of the brain adenyl cyclase system. Vol. 3, p. 11–30. In: P. Greengard and E. Costa (Eds.). Role of Cyclic AMP in Cell Function. Advances in Biochemical Psychopharmacology, New York: Raven Press 1970

Rosenblum, W.I.: Control of cerebral blood flow by pial arterioles. 50th Annual Meeting of the American Association of Neuropathologists, Boston, 1974

Rosenfeld, E.L.: Animal tissue γ-amylase and its rôle in the meabolism of glycogen, p. 176–182. In: W.J. Wheelan and M.P. Cameron (Eds.). Control of Glycogen Metabolism. London: Churchill 1964

Rothenberg, M.A.: Studies on permeability in relation to nerve function. II. Ionic movements across axonal membranes. Biochim. Biophys. Acta. **4**, 96–114 (1950)

Rottenberg, D.A., Passonneau, J.V., Lust, W.D.: Glycogen-mediated activation of pig-brain glycogen synthetase I and D, Biochem. biophys. Res. Commun. **48**, 1192–1198 (1972)

Samson, M.: Serotonine et système nerveux central. J. Path. Biol. **12**, 1102–1106 (1964)

Sasaki, M., Takeuchi, T.: Histochemical and electron microscopic observations of glycogen synthesized from glucose-l-phosphate by phosphorylase and branching enzyme in human muscle. J. Histochem. Cytochem. **11**, 342–348 (1963)

Sasse, D.: Untersuchungen zur nachweismethodik der Uridindiphosphoglukose-glycogen-transferase. Histochemie, **7**, 39–49 (1966)

Sawyer, D., Sie, H., Fishman, W.H., A technique for preparing permanent histochemical preparations of liver phosphorylase. J. Histochem. Cytochem. **13**, 605–607 (1965)

Schabadasch, A.L.: Morphology of glycogen distribution and transformations. III. Cytology of glycogen accumulations in the motor cells of the normal nervous system. Bull. Biol. med. exp. **7**, 353–357 (1939)

Schmidt, M. J., Schmidt, D. E., Robison, G. A.: Cyclic adenosine monophosphate in brain areas: Microwave irradiation as a means of tissue fixation. Science **173**, 1142–1143 (1971)

Schneider, H., Dralle, J.: Ultrastructural changes in the rat spinal cord after temporary occlusion of the thoracic aorta. Acta neuropathol. (Berl.), **26**, 301–315 (1973)

Schuberth, J., Sollenberg, J., Sundwall, A., Sörbo, B.: Acetyl-coenzyme A in brain. The effect of centrally active drugs, insulin coma and hypoxia. J. Neurochem. **13**, 819–822 (1966)

Schultz, J., Daly, J. W.: Adenosine-3′,5′-monophosphate in guinea pig cerebral cortical slices: Effects of α- and β-adrenergic agents, histamine, serotonin and adenosine. J. Neurochem. **21**, 573–579 (1973)

Selinger, Z., Schramm, M.: An insoluble complex formed by the interaction of muscle phosphorylase with glycogen. Biochem. biophys. Res. Commun. **12**, 208–214 (1963)

Shanthaveerappa, T. R., Waitzman, M. B., Bourne, G. H.: Studies on the distribution of phosphorylase in eyes of the rabbit and the squirrel monkey. Histochemie **7**, 80–95 (1966)

Shimazu, T.: Glycogen synthetase activity in liver: Regulation by the autonomic nerves. Science **156**, 1256–1257 (1967)

Shimizu, H., Creveling, C. R., Daly, J. W.: Effect of membrane depolarization and biogenic amines on the formation cyclic AMP in incubated brain slices. Vol. 3, p. 135–154. In: P. Greengard and E. Costo (Eds.). Rôle of cyclic AMP in Cell Function. Advances in Biochemical Psychopharmacology. New York: Raven Press 1970

Shimizu, H., Tanaka, S., Suzuki, T., Matsukado, Y.: The response of human cerebrum adenyl cyclase to biogenic amines. J. Neurochem. **18**, 1157–1161 (1971)

Shimizu, N. A.: A histochemical investigation on the brain glycogen of rabbits with elevated blood-glucose. Wakayama Igaku (in Japanese) **5**, 9–12 (1954). Cited by Friede, R. L. Topographic Brain Chemistry. p. 142. New York: Academic Press 1966

Shimizu, N. A., Hamuro, Y.: Deposition of glycogen and changes in some enzymes in brain wounds. Nature (Lond.) **181**, 781–782 (1958)

Shimizu, N. A., Kubo, Z.: Histochemical studies on brain glycogen of the guinea pig and its alteration following electric shock. J. Neuropathol. exp. Neurol. **16**, 40–47 (1957)

Shimizu, N. A., Kumamoto, T.: Histochemical studies on the glycogen of the mammalian brain. Anat. Rec. **114**, 479–497 (1952)

Shimizu, N. A., Maeda, S.: Histochemical studies on glycogen of the retina. Anat. Rec. **116**, 427–437 (1953)

Shimizu, N., Okada, M.: Histochemical distribution of phosphorylase in rodent brain from newborn to adults. J. Histochem. Cytochem. **5**, 459–471 (1957)

Shiraki, H.: The comparative study of various types of hepatocerebral diseases in the Japanese, p. 252. In: O. T. Bailey and D. E. Smith (Eds.). The Central Nervous System. Baltimore: Williams and Wilkins 1958

Shtark, M. B.: Histochemistry of glycogen in the encephalon of hybernating animals, Dokl. Akad. Nauk SSSR (Physiol.), **153**, 1216–1220 (1963). Cited by R. L. Friede: Topographic Brain Chemistry, p. 142. New York: Academic Press 1966

Sie, H. G., Hablanian, A., Fishman, W. H.: Solubilization of mouse liver glycogen synthetase and phosphorylase during starvation glycogenolysis and its reversal by cortisol. Nature (Lond.) **201**, 393–394 (1964)

Sie, H. G., Sawyer, D., Fishman, W. H.: Enzymorphologic demonstration of glucose-6-phosphate-dependent glycogen synthetase in mouse liver. J. Histochem. Cytochem. **14**, 247–253 (1966)

Simeone, F. A., Ryan, K. G., Cotter, J. R.: Prolonged experimental cerebral vasospasm. J. Neurosurg. **29**, 357–366 (1968)

Sjöstrand, J.: Changes in nucleoside phosphatase activity in the hypoglossal nucleus during nerve regeneration. Acta physiol. scand. **67**, 219–228 (1966a)

Sjöstrand, J.: Studies on glial cells in the hypoglossal nucleus of the rabbit during nerve regeneration. Acta physiol. scand. **67** (suppl. 270), 2–17 (1966b)

Skoff, R. P., Price, D. L.: Proliferation of reactive astrocytes in degenerating rat optic nerve. 50th Annual Meeting of the American Association of Neuropathologists, Boston. 1974

Skoff, R. P., Vaughn, J. E.: An autoradiographic study of cellular proliferation in degenerating rat optic nerve. J. comp. Neurol. **141**, 133–156 (1971)

Skolnick, P., Huang, M., Daly, J., Hoffer, B.: Accumulation of adenosine-3′,5′-monophosphate in incubated slices from discrete regions of squirrel monkey cerebral cortex: effect of norepenephrine, serotonin and adenosine. J. Neurochem. **21**, 237–240 (1973)

Śmialek, M., Sikorska, M., Bicz, W., Mossakowski, M. J.: UDP glucose: glycogen α-4-glucosyl-transferase (EC 2.4.1.11) and α-1,4-glucan: orthophosphate glucosyltransferase (E.C. 2.4.1.1) activity in rat brain in experimental ischaemia. Acta neuropathol. (Berl.) 19, 242–248 (1971)

Śmialek, M., Sikorska, M., Korthals, J., Bicz, W., Mossakowski, M. J.: The glycogen content and its topography and UDP glucose: glycogen α-4 glucosyltransferase (E.C. 2.4.1.11) activity in rat brain after experimental carbon monoxide intoxication. Acta neuropathol. (Berl.) 24, 222–231 (1973)

Smith, A. A.: Histochemical differentiation of two forms of glycogen synthetase. J. Histochem. Cytochem. 18, 756–759 (1970)

Smith, A. A., Perkins, E. M., Machida, H.: Durable mounts of the iodine stain for the phosphorylase reaction. Stain Technol. 41, 346–348 (1966)

Smith, K. R., Jr., Hudgens, R. W., O'Leary, J. L.: An electron microscopic study of degenerative changes in the cat cerebellum after intrinsic and extrinsic lesions. J. comp. Neurol. 126, 15–36 (1966)

Smitherman, M. L., Lazarow, A., Sorenson, R. L.: The effect of light microscopic fixatives on the retention of glycogen in protein matrices and the particulate state of native glycogen. J. Histochem. Cytochem. 20, 463–471 (1972)

Sommerville, A. R., Smith, A. A.: The effects of propranolol and electrical stimulation on the cyclic -3',5'-AMP content of isolated cerebral tissue. J. Neurochem. 19, 2003–2006 (1972)

Sotelo, C., Wegmann, R.: Différences du métabolisme des glucides de la substance blanche et de la substance grise du cervelet. Acta histochem. (Jena) 18, 125–136 (1964)

Spector, R. G.: Water content of the brain in anoxic-ischaemic encephalopathy in adult rats. Brit. J. exp. Path. 42, 623–630 (1961)

Spector, W., Willoughby, D.: 5-Hydroxytryptamine in acute inflammation. Nature (Lond.) 179, 318 (1957)

Steiner, D., Younger, L., King, J.: Purification and properties of uridine diphosphate glucose-glycogen glucosyltransferase from rat liver. Biochemistry (Wash.) 4, 740–751 (1965)

Stetten, D., Jr., Stetten, M. R.: Glycogen metabolism. Physiol. Rev. 40, 505–537 (1960)

Stewart, M. A., Moonsammy, G. I.: Substrate changes in peripheral nerve recovering from anoxia. J. Neurochem. 13, 1433–1439 (1966)

Stewart, M. A., Passonneau, J. V., Lowry, O. H.: Substrate changes in peripheral nerve during ischaemia and Wallerian degeneration. J. Neurochem. 12, 719–727 (1965)

Stewart, M. A., Sherman, W. R., Kurien, M. M., Moonsammy, G. I., Wisgerhof, M.: Polyol accumulations in nervous tissue of rats with experimental diabetes and galactosaemia. J. Neurochem. 14, 1057–1066 (1967)

Sutherland, E. W.: Studies on the mechanism of hormone action. Science 177, 401–408 (1972)

Sutherland, E. W., Rall, T. W.: The relation of adenosine-3',5'-phosphate and phosphorylase to the actions of catecholamines and other hormones. Pharmacol. Rev. 12, 265–299 (1960)

Sutherland, E. W., Wosilait, W. D.: The relationship of epinephrine and glucagon to liver phosphorylase. (I) Liver phosphorylase; preparation and properties. J. biol. Chem. 218, 459–468 (1956)

Svorad, D.: Changes in the topographic distribution of glycogen in the brain during animal hypnosis. Nature (Lond.) 181, 775–776 (1958)

Swanson, M. A.: Studies on the structure of polysaccharides. (IV) Relation of the iodine color to the structure. J. biol. Chem. 172, 825–837 (1948)

Swigart, R. H., Wagner, C. E., Atkinson, W. B.: The preservation of glycogen in fixed tissues and tissue sections, J. Histochem. Cytochem. 8, 74–75 (1960)

Szentágothai, J., Hámori, J., Tömböl, T.: Degeneration and electron microscope analysis of the synaptic glomeruli in the lateral geniculate body. Exp. Brain Res. 2, 283–301 (1966)

Takei, Y., Solitare, G. B.: Infantile spongy degeneration of the central nervous system associated with glycogen storage and markedly fatty liver. J. Neurol. Neurosurg. Psychiatr. 35, 11–21 (1972)

Takeuchi, T.: Histochemical demonstration of phosphorylase. J. Histochem. Cytochem. 4, 84 (1956)

Takeuchi, T.: Histochemical demonstration of branching enzyme (amylo-1,4→1,6-transglucosidase) in animal tissues. J. Histochem. Cytochem. 6, 208–216 (1958)

Takeuchi, T.: Histochemical demonstration of phosphorylase in nerve tissues. J. Histochem. Cytochem. 13, 722 (1965a)

Takeuchi, T.: Histochemical observation of glycogen metabolism in nerve tissues. Recent Advances in Research of the Nervous System. (in Japanese) 9, 695–699 (1965 b)

Takeuchi, T.: Electron microscopic differences between native glycogen and polyglucose histochemically synthesized by enzymes in rabbit skeletal muscles. J. Histochem. Cytochem. 18, 687 (1970)

Takeuchi, T., Glenner, G. G.: Histochemical demonstration of uridine diphosphate glucose-glycogen transferase in animal tissues. J. Histochem. Cytochem. 9, 304–316 (1961)

Takeuchi, T., Higashi, K., Watanuki, S.: Distribution of amylophosphorylase in various tissues of human and mammalian organs. J. Histochem. Cytochem. 3, 485–491 (1955)

Takeuchi, T., Kuriaki, H.: Histochemical detection of phosphorylase in animal tissue. J. Histochem. Cytochem. 3, 153–160 (1955)

Takeuchi, T., Sasaki, M.: Validity of the histochemical phosphorylase and uridine diphosphate-glycogen transglucosylase methods. J. Histochem. Cytochem. 18, 761–765 (1970)

Tata, J.R.: Subcellular redistribution of liver α-glucan phosphorylase during alterations in glycogen content. Biochem. J. 90, 284–292 (1964)

Tews, J.K., Carter, S.H., Stone, W.E.: Chemical changes in the brain during insulin hypoglycaemia and recovery. J. Neurochem. 12, 679–693 (1965)

Thorn, W., Isselhard, W., Müldener, B.: Glykogen-, Glucose- und Milchsauregehalt in Warmblüterorganen bei unterschiedlicher Versuchsanordnung und anoxischer Belastung mit Hilfe optischer Fermentteste ermittelt. Biochem. Z. 331, 545–562 (1959)

Thurston, J.H., Pierce, R.W.: Increase of glucose and high energy phosphate reserve in the brain after hydrocortisone. J. Neurochem. 16, 107–111 (1969)

Timiras, P.S., Woodbury, D.M., Baker, D.H.: Effect of hydrocortisone acetate, desoxycorticosterone acetate, insulin, glucagon and dextrose, alone or in combination, on experimental convulsions and carbohydrate metabolism. Arch. int. Pharmacodyn. 105, 450–467 (1956)

Torack, R.M.: Electron histochemistry of the nervous system. In: C.W.M. Adams (Ed.), p. 167. Neurohistochemistry. Amsterdam: Elsevier 1965

Tourtellotte, W.W., Lowry, O.H., Passonneau, J.V., O'Leary, J.L., Harris, A.B., Rowe, III J.J.: Carbohydrate metabolites in rabbit hereditary ataxia. Arch. Neurol. (Chic.) 15, 283–288 (1966)

Trufanov, A.V., Popova, G.M.: Biosynthesis of coenzyme A by tissue homogenates, Biokhimiya 21, 1–6 (1956)

Tsukada, Y., Takaguchi, G.: Effect of potassium ions on brain slices. Nature (Lond.) 175, 725–726 (1955)

Vaccari, F., Malaguti, G.: Boll. Soc. ital. Biol. sper. 27, 1627 (1951). Cited by Thurston, J.H. and Pierce, R.W. Increase of glucose and high energy phosphate reserve in the brain after hydrocortisone. J. Neurochem. 16, 107–111 (1969)

Veloso, D., Passonneau, J.V., Veech, R.L.: The effects of intoxicating doses of ethanol upon intermediary metabolism in rat brain, J. Neurochem. 19, 2679–2686 (1972)

Vigh-Teichmann, I., Vigh, B.: The infundibular cerebrospinal-fluid containing neurons. Adv. Anat. Embryol. and Cell Biol. Vol. 50, Fasc. 2. Berlin-Heidelberg-New York: Springer 1974

Villar-Palasi, C., Larner, J.: Glycogen metabolism and glycolytic enzymes. Ann. Rev. Biochem. 39, 639–672 (1970)

Wanson, J.-C., Drochmans, P.: Rabbit skeletal muscle glycogen. A morphological and biochemical study of glycogen β-particles isolated by the precepitation-centrifugation method. J. Cell Biol. 38, 130–150 (1968)

Watanabe, H., Passonneau, J.V.: Factors affecting the turnover of cerebral glycogen and limit dextrin in vivo. J. Neurochem. 20, 1543–1554 (1973)

Watanabe, I., Patel, V., Goebel, H.H., Siakotos, A.N., Zeman, W., Meyer, W.De, Dyer, J.S.: Early lesion of Pelizaeus-Merzbacher disease: electron microscopic and biochemical study. J. Neuropathol. exp. Neurol. 32, 313–333 (1973)

Wegmann, R., Sotelo, C.: Systemes metaboliques coordonnes pour l'etude enzymologique du systeme nerveux. Arch. belg. Dermatol. Syphiligr. 19, 335–350 (1963)

Welch, K.M.A., Hashi, K., Meyer, J.S.: Cerebrovascular response to intracarotid injection of serotonin before and after middle cerebral artery occlusion. J. Neurol. Neurosurg. Psychiatr. 36, 724–735 (1973)

Wesemann, I., Kuss, B., Breurer, H., Parchwitz, H.K.: Wirkung einer Röntgenbestrahlung auf den Glukose- und Fettsäuretransport im Dünndarm der Ratte. Strahlentherapie 119, 425–434 (1962)

West, E.S., Todd, W.R., Mason, H.S., Van Bruggen, J.T.: Textbook of Biochemistry. 4th Ed., p. 1064. New York: The Macmillan 1966

Willougby, D.A.: Pharmacological aspects of the vascular permeability changes in the rat's intestine following abdominal radiation. Brit. J. Radiol. 33, 515–519 (1960)

Wittels, B.: Myocardial glycogen in the fetus, infant and child. Arch. Path. 75, 127–138 (1963)

Wolff, H.: Histochemische und Elektronenmikroskopische Beobachtungen über die Glykogenverteilung in Hypothalamus einiger Winterschläfer (Mit quantitativen Bemerkungen). Z. Zellforsch. 88, 228–261 (1968)

Wurtzman, R.J., Zervas, N.T.: Monoamine neurotransmitters and the pathophysiology of stroke and central nervous system trauma. J. Neurosurg. 40, 34–36 (1974)

Yin, H.C., Sun, C.N.: Histochemical method for the detection of phosphorylase in plant tissues. Science 105, 650 (1947)

Yu, M.C., Bakay, L., Lee, J.C.: Ultrastructure of the central nervous system after prolonged hypoxia. I. Neuronal alterations. Acta neuropathol. (Berl.) 22, 222–234 (1972a)

Yu, M.C., Bakay, L., Lee, J.C.: Ultrastructure of the central nervous system after prolonged hypoxia. II. Neuroglia and blood vessels. Acta neuropathol. (Berl.) 22, 235–244 (1972b)

Zeman, W.: Histochemical and metabolic changes in brain tissue after hypoxaemia. p. 327–348. In: J.P. Schadé and W.H. McMenemey (Eds.). Selective Vulnerability of the Brain in Hypoxaemia. Philadelphia: Davis 1963

Subject Index

85